Advance Praise for *The IBD Healing Plan and Recipe Book*

"Christie Korth's new book is a breath of fresh air among the many books that have the same old stale information. Knowing Christie and working with her, I am continually impressed by the depth of her knowledge and her ability to relate it to others in a practical way. This book reveals cutting-edge information presented in a fun, entertaining, and compassionate way. You can tell that her primary goal is to give the best information possible and to help suffering people. Christie's personal story is an inspiration to us all and should inspire the reader as well. I strongly recommend this book to anyone not only with IBD but with any chronic illness."

— Dr. Robert Melillo, Author of *Disconnected Kids and Reconnected Kids,*
Co-founder of Brain Balance Achievement Centers,
Executive Director of The FR Carrick Research Institute
and Children's Autism Hope Project,
President of the International Association of
Functional Neurology and Rehabilitation,
Co-editor of the *Journal of Functional Neurology,
Rehabilitation and Ergonomics*

"Christie's personal and interactive approach, combined with a wealth of well-researched information, is the perfect guide to help you take control of your own health and well-being. She helps you navigate the mountain of misleading dietary information out there and find health and happiness through food and lifestyle changes."

— Joshua Rosenthal, MSEd, Author of *Integrative Nutrition,*
Founder, Professor, and Director of
The Institute for Integrative Nutrition of NYC

"During the past decade a holistic approach to nutrition has become more recognized as a valid approach to managing various medical disorders. Gone are the days when food was just something to fill the bellies of the children and drugs alone were the only option when they got sick. Food has finally come of age as an integral part of natural medicine.

Christie Korth's *The IBD Healing Plan and Recipe Book* is an important work that I believe will further bring holistic nutrition to individuals needing care in this area.

Besides being a doctor, I am also a *cancer survivor*. I used holistic nutrition on myself, as well as traditional treatments, to improve my own health situation. So I know firsthand how nutrition can help the body heal.

I've been waiting for a book like this to come along to bring this knowledge to a wider audience.

Ms. Korth's book fulfills its mission in two ways. First, [it includes] inspiring stories of people who were afraid that the traditional approaches to handling their health conditions would leave them physically and psychologically damaged but were able to manage their conditions nutritionally and live happy, productive lives.

Second, Ms. Korth offers a variety of recipes and shopping tips that will help readers maintain a tasty diet while managing their condition.

Furthermore, the book is an easy read. I'm sure readers will agree, its combination of stories, recipes, and advice will result in a pleasant reading experience. This is a book all can digest and enjoy.

— Dr. Robert J. Lichtenstein, DC, CNS
Chiropractic physician
Board-certified Nutrition Specialist

"Christie's experience and insight—both personally and professionally, working with clients who have IBD—combined with her practical no-nonsense manner of dealing with the nutritional challenges of these disorders make her book a must-read for anyone suffering with IBD.

Her book is fun, interactive, and written in a manner that any person can comprehend and put into practical use on a daily basis."

— Philip J. Antz, LCSW

Ordering
Trade bookstores in the U.S. and Canada please contact
Publishers Group West
1700 Fourth St., Berkeley CA 94710
Phone: (800) 788-3123   Fax: (800) 351-5073

For bulk orders please contact
Special Sales
Hunter House Inc., PO Box 2914, Alameda CA 94501-0914
Phone: (510) 899-5041   Fax: (510) 865-4295
E-mail: sales@hunterhouse.com

Individuals can order our books by calling **(800) 266-5592**
or from our website at **www.hunterhouse.com**

The
IBD
Healing Plan
and Recipe Book

USING WHOLE FOODS
TO RELIEVE
CROHN'S DISEASE
AND COLITIS

CHRISTIE A. KORTH, CHC, AADP

Hunter House PUBLISHERS

Hunter House Inc., Publishers
PO Box 2914
Alameda CA 94501-0914

Library of Congress Cataloging-in-Publication Data
Korth, Christie A.
The IBD healing plan and recipe book : using whole foods to relieve
Crohn's disease and colitis / Christie A. Korth. — 1st ed.
p. cm.
Includes bibliographical references and index.
ISBN 978-0-89793-612-5 (pbk.)
ISBN 978-0-89793-613-2 (ebk.)
1. Inflammatory bowel diseases — Diet therapy. 2. Inflammatory bowel
diseases — Diet therapy — Recipes. 3. Inflammatory bowel diseases —
Psychological aspects. I. Title.
RC862.I53K68 2012
616.3'44 — dc23   2012019225

Project Credits

Cover Design: Jinni Fontana

Book Production: John McKercher

Illustrator: Bijal Gosalia

Photographers: John Korth and
Angelica Korth

Developmental Editor: Jude Berman

Copy Editor: Heather Wilcox

Reviewer: Jessica Hurley

Proofreader: Lori Cavanaugh

Indexers: Robert and Cynthia Swanson

Managing Editor: Alexandra Mummery

Acquisitions Assistant: Elana Fiske

Special Sales Manager: Judy Hardin

Rights Coordinator:
Candace Groskreutz

Customer Service Manager:
Christina Sverdrup

Order Fulfillment: Washul Lakdhon

Administrator: Theresa Nelson

IT Support: Peter Eichelberger

Publisher: Kiran S. Rana

Printed and bound by Sheridan Books, Ann Arbor, Michigan
Manufactured in the United States of America

9 8 7 6 5 4 3 2   First Edition   13 14 15 16 17

Contents

Foreword ix

Acknowledgments xi

Introduction 1
   My Story 1
   My Approach 5
   My Mission 6

1 Inflammatory Bowel Disease 101 7
   Stephanie's Story 8
   The IBD Family 11
   Who Gets IBD? 13
   The Science Behind IBD 14
   Common Treatment Methods Used in Western Medicine 15
   Why a Holistic Approach? 17
   Working on Your Primary Health Puzzle Pieces to Manage IBD . 18
   The American Lifestyle and a Holistic Approach to Disease . . . 19
   How Can Blue Zones Teach You about Holistic Health? 22
   IBD Medications and Nutritional Deficiencies 26
   How to Adopt a Holistic Lifestyle: Making Positive Changes . . . 28
   Take a Stand—Change Your Digestion! 29
   Food for Thought 34

2 Food Intolerance and Inflammatory Bowel Disease 36
   Frank's Story 37
   Food Intolerance and IBD 38
   Understanding Your Immune System 39
   Food Addiction, Leaky Gut Syndrome, and IgG Reactions 44
   Common Sensitivities 46

The Top Eight Allergens 46
Food Intolerance and Proteins 46
The Science Behind IBD and Food Intolerance 50
Testing Methods for Food Intolerance. 56
The Food Diary 56
The Digestion Diary. 57
The Food-Elimination Diet. 63
The Reintroduction Diet 65
The Rotation Diet. 69
Grocery Shopping Cards 71

3 Now That I Know I Have IBD, Which Foods Can Affect Me?

Now That I Know I Have IBD, Which Foods
Can Affect Me? 81
Steve's Story. 81
Food Politics 83
Back to Nature: Organics 101. 86
Sugar and IBD 90
Caffeine Consumption and IBD 97
Tips for Kicking the Caffeine Habit 99

4 Soothing Foods for the Intestines

Soothing Foods for the Intestines 100
Michael's Story 100
Anti-Inflammatory Foods 101
Fruits and Vegetables. 102
Whole Grains 106
Essential Fatty Acids 107
IBD and the Vegetarian/Vegan Diet 108
Put It All Together. 111
Healthy Anti-Inflammatory Lunch Ideas for Those on the Go . . 113

5 Establishing a Supplement Regime for Inflammatory Bowel Disease

Establishing a Supplement Regime
for Inflammatory Bowel Disease. 115
Daphne's Story. 115
Supplements for a Special Digestive System 117
Nature's Painkillers 126

6 Essential IBD Resources

Essential IBD Resources 129
Tiffany's Story 129
Eating for Your Blood Type 130
Your Menu Planner 133

Sample Allergen-Free Menu 135

Mindful Eating 136

To Sum It Up 140

7 The Recipe Corner 143

Erick's Story 143

A Note Regarding the Nutritional Information in the Recipes . . 144

A Note Regarding Organic Foods 144

A Note Regarding Healthy Fish, Meat, and Poultry 145

Breakfast 146

Smoothies and Beverages 163

Appetizers and Snack Foods 175

Soups 183

Beans 187

Meat and Poultry 191

Fish 203

Grains and Pasta 208

Vegetables 216

Salads 227

Snacks and Desserts 233

Dressings, Sauces, and Dips 248

Notes 256

Resources 263

Index 267

*Dedicated to my little Bear, Jayden, and my sweet baby Pea.
I love you both more than there are waves in the ocean,
grains of sand on the beach, and stars in the sky.*

*Jayden Michael, you are the most special person in my life,
and I could not ask for a more loving, beautiful,
or intelligent little boy. You are my little hero,
my inspiration, and miracle.*

*My Pea, I am thankful that even if for only a short while,
you shared your soul with mine. You have both taught me
the greatest lessons in life and are the driving force
pushing me to do amazing things.*

*The Lord has blessed me beyond infinity to be your mother,
and for that I am eternally grateful.*

With all my love, Mama

Important Note

The material in this book is intended to provide a review of information regarding inflammatory bowel disease (IBD). Every effort has been made to provide accurate and dependable information. The contents of this book have been compiled through professional research and in consultation with medical professionals. However, health-care professionals have differing opinions, and advances in medical and scientific research are made very quickly, so some of the information may become outdated.

Therefore, the publisher, authors, and editors, as well as the professionals quoted in the book, cannot be held responsible for any error, omission, or dated material. The authors and publisher assume no responsibility for any outcome of applying the information in this book in a program of self-care or under the care of a licensed practitioner. If you have questions concerning your nutrition or diet, or about the application of the information described in this book, consult a qualified health-care professional.

Foreword

There is much truth in the old adage "You are what you eat," and although science has taught us that dietary intake is only one piece of the wellness puzzle, I have come to believe that it is one of the most important. While none of us has the ability to change our pasts, our family medical histories, or our genetics, we do have the power to control what we put into our bodies.

Because the foods we consume can profoundly affect our overall health and well-being, the astounding number of people suffering from inflammatory bowel disease and digestive tract disorders should not come as a surprise. We live in a culture filled with overprocessed, contaminated, prepackaged convenience foods that are making us sicker than ever before.

Most people know someone suffering from illnesses such as Crohn's disease, ulcerative colitis, irritable bowel syndrome, and acid reflux. Perhaps you were diagnosed with one of these disorders and know firsthand how the painful symptoms and constant fear of flare-ups can prohibit you from living the life you want.

Over the past decade, many individuals have become more health conscious and try to make the "right" choices. But when constantly bombarded with advice on what to eat, what to avoid, and conflicting information on the latest and greatest "super foods," it has become increasingly difficult to make sense of it all.

What many people do not realize is that an entire industry of health professionals is dedicated to providing the most reliable, up-to-date nutritional information available. Dieticians, nutritionists, and holistic-health counselors specialize in wellness through dietary change and can help you sift through the information and generalized confusion.

Christie Korth is one of these professionals. She has written a smart, commonsense book packed with information, worksheets, self-assessment tools, and recipes to aid those suffering from inflammatory bowel disease in making positive lifestyle changes.

I have the pleasure of working with Christie on a weekly basis. The depth of her knowledge regarding foods, vitamins, and minerals and how they can help the body heal is tremendous. As a health-care practitioner specializing in pain management, I have come to appreciate the use of multiple modalities in treating my patients. I have also learned not to underestimate the impact that nutritional status has on overall health. I confidently refer patients from my practice to Christie and have consistently witnessed the improvements of those who have undergone her nutritional counseling.

Many years of experience have lead Christie to focus on food intolerances. Unlike food allergies, which can cause redness, swelling, rashes, and respiratory difficulty, the outward effects of food intolerance can be hard to recognize. Because most of us are unaware of our dietary intolerances, we continue to assault our system with the same foods that are making us sick, and the effects on our digestive tract can be devastating. Repetitive exposure to these items can lead to chronic irritation, inflammation, and immune reactions that have a negative effect on our total wellness.

Fortunately, *The IBD Healing Plan and Recipe Book* provides access to the professional nutritional counseling that so many of us desperately need. You will find the expert guidance needed to assess your individual food intolerances, along with specific methods to end the destructive behaviors that keep you unhealthy. This book provides the necessary tools to free yourself from the confines of intestinal tract disorders.

I am privileged to know Christie as a colleague and as a friend, and I am excited by the knowledge that this book has the ability to empower its readers to improve their health, to end their suffering from inflammatory bowel disease, and to bring about positive change in their lives!

— Christie Petras, PA-C
Physician's assistant

Acknowledgments

First and foremost, I am very thankful to God for allowing me the opportunity to help others by sharing my own experience, expertise, and knowledge. Writing a book is something that I have aspired to do since childhood, somehow always knowing deep down that I would be an author. It is priceless to have written my first book about a topic that is so close to my heart. Without my faith in Him, none of this would have been possible.

I live my life practicing the law of attraction. Due to this belief system, I understand that nothing in life is coincidental. Each time a perceived "coincidence" comes my way, I am more motivated to keep plowing forward on my life's mission. I must acknowledge a particular day that occurred as I was finishing this manuscript. My parents had called to alert me of a flood in their basement. Upon arriving to check out the damage, I was horrified: The flood was quite extensive, and the crumbling sheetrock had fallen from the walls, leaving large slabs of concrete exposed. It was there, in blue crayon, I discovered my very own eight-year-old handwriting. In sloppy, block lettering, it read, "Heal the world, make it a better place..." and all of the lyrics to Michael Jackson's song, "Heal the World" followed. In the midst of such devastation, a chill crept up my spine when I realized the "coincidence" of the timing.

I couldn't help but wonder whether the younger me knew I would grow up to be a nutritionist who tries to "heal the world," one person at a time. I am truly living out my life-long dream. This book is a manifestation of a vision to help others who suffer from Crohn's or colitis, as I once did. For this opportunity, I am immensely blessed and grateful.

I thank the staff at Hunter House for their insight and guidance and for allowing me to fulfill my dream by printing this manuscript.

I would also like to thank Bayu, who helped me figure out what was causing my Crohn's disease. Without him, I would still be sick, and we wouldn't have our beautiful son, Jayden Michael—or this book. To the angel of a woman who told me while in the hospital to read *Patient Heal Thyself*, which I firmly believe saved my life—I don't know who you are, but you not only helped me, you changed my life. God bless you. And of course, thank you to Mom, who was by my side through the worst of my "sick" days, and to Dad, who instilled a love for nutrition when I was a child and taught me the importance of positive thinking. Thank you to my siblings along with my dearest friends, Raymond, Tiffany, and Jen, for continuing to stick by me, no matter what.

I would also like to acknowledge my mentors, Dr. Robert Lichtenstein, Dr. Bill Akpinar, Dr. Robert Melillo, Phillip Antz, and Christine Petras. I am so grateful to work alongside so many wonderfully caring, dynamic professionals. You each have motivated me to tap into my unlimited potential by being exemplary beacons in your fields. I am beyond thankful to the staff at Integrated for allowing me to be part of a practice that complements modern medicine with nutrition and other holistic practices. Thank you for continuing to teach me and help me grow as a practitioner by expanding my knowledge base.

To my Brain Balance Family for their continued support, encouragement, and professional alliance: You are all the best! Being a part of the BB atmosphere inspires me every day to become better at what I do to help others. To my top-notch staff at my practice, Happy & Healthy Wellness—no words for you guys except "amazing." Thank you for helping me spread happiness and healthiness far and wide and for fulfilling my dream to have a thriving practice. And last, but certainly not least, to my clients: You give me back the greatest gift, watching people bask in the glow of health. Thank you for allowing me to have the best job under the sun.

Introduction

Before I was diagnosed with Crohn's disease at age nineteen, I had never even heard of the debilitating condition that would change my life. I was clueless, knowing absolutely nothing about it. Times have changed! These days, I possess so much information on the topic I'm like a walking Crohn's and colitis encyclopedia!

It is likely that if you are reading this book, you or a loved one is suffering from inflammatory bowel disease (IBD). I invite you to read about my very own healing journey, mission, and purpose for writing it. I have dedicated my career to helping people with IBD, and I hope that *The IBD Healing Plan and Recipe Book* will be the first step in your personal healing journey.

My Story

Not too long ago, illness had virtually consumed my life. For as far back as I could remember, my childhood had been plagued by a mysterious, tremendous stomach pain. When I turned nine, my mother grew concerned and dragged me around from doctor to doctor, trying to find the root cause of my excruciating symptoms.

Despite all of the tests that I endured, the results were not conclusive. Colonoscopy and endoscopy results were normal, with the exception of an ulcer. I didn't know any other nine-year-olds with an ulcer. I had gotten to the point where I would actually pray that doctors would find something else wrong, with the sound reasoning that if they found the cause, then *someone* would know how to fix it. My traditional German pediatrician, who was not into prescribing meds, was at her wits' end. She thought dairy intolerance was to blame, but alas, my stomach still hurt even after *months* on Lactaid milk and an entire summer foregoing the ice cream truck. When this theory was proven incorrect, I moved on to daily scheduled dosages of antacid medications, along with Mylanta and Pepto-Bismol. As a last resort, Mom even took me to a counselor, suspecting stress was to blame for my ailments. But this cause was also ruled out, because I was a pretty happy, well-adjusted kid. At that point, I sort of gave up all hope of finding a diagnosis and chalked up my symptoms to having a "sensitive" stomach.

I managed as best as I could until things took a frightening turn when I started college. I was five feet six inches tall, but I lost about 20 pounds in two short months, dropping from a healthy 130 pounds to a gaunt 110 pounds. I could not eat without desperately needing a bathroom almost immediately afterward due to diarrhea. One of my professors even expressed concern, wondering why I often left class to use the restroom. The straw that broke the camel's back was the onset of recurring bleeding episodes (blood in my stool). I knew something was very wrong at that point. I decided to look for a diagnosis again and made an appointment with a new gastroenterologist.

It had been ten years of tests, misdiagnoses, medications, and missed school days, and I was finally diagnosed with Crohn's disease, an inflammatory bowel disease (IBD) that affects the small intestine. I was nineteen years old and completely confounded by the diagnosis.

I had always believed that once I discovered my symptoms were attached to an actual illness, I would finally get better. An effective treatment protocol must exist, right?

To my horror, it seemed that no matter what medications my doctor prescribed, my disease didn't seem to improve at all. In fact, it was only getting worse, despite the fact that I had tried each and every medical option available. I couldn't eat without vomiting afterward, and I spent most of my time cooped up in a bathroom. I had no more meds to try, because I had already been on all of them, including Remicade infusions and 6MP. I was *really* at the end of my rope.

I got so sick that I became a prisoner in my house. I never knew when a flare-up would occur, so I avoided going out whenever I didn't absolutely have to. Ultimately, becoming a hermit led to the lowest point of my life. Reluctantly, I took a leave of absence from college and my job. I was in disbelief. If I had a diagnosis, why didn't any of the prescribed treatments work? Some of them seemed to have made me feel even *worse*. For instance, when I was prescribed steroids, my blood sugar would drop prior to mealtimes. I would become so agitated that I felt the need to actually *avoid* people for fear of biting their heads off. I was desperately hungry *all* of the time! What a scary reaction! I lived like this for three years, on and off different medications and in and out of the hospital. All the while, I strived to remain positive while praying for a miracle.

And boy, did I get one. When I was twenty-two, I was admitted to the hospital for yet another Crohn's flare-up. I was experiencing a 104°F fever, severe vomiting, and relentless trips to the bathroom. The pain was unbearable. My doctors told me that if I didn't have my intestines removed, I would die. Oddly enough, all fear became consumed by a fierce focus. I was determined to make it out of the hospital with my intestines intact and *without* a colostomy bag. I refused to settle for less.

I started telling my hospital roommate about my plight. She then told me about the book *Patient Heal Thyself*, by Jordan Rubin. The book discusses Rubin's own harrowing ordeal with Crohn's. The author had studied primitive ways of eating from the Bible to harness the power of nutrition and digestion, and he eventually healed himself. My roommate claimed that this book had saved a dear friend of hers from the effects of the disease that was crippling me.

After hearing that there was possibly another way I could get well, I knew I had no choice but to give it a shot: It was that or lose my intestines. I resisted doctors' warnings, including a potentially fatal prognosis, and left the hospital against medical advice. Please understand that I do *not* recommend that you follow my path here. My decision to leave the hospital sounds radical and irrational, and it was. I cannot describe the feeling that came over me. A surgeon was on his way to my room to discuss taking out my insides, and I simply could not even bear the thought. My family and friends pleaded with me to stay. My husband and I were dating at the time, and I begged him to bring me home. He obliged, despite obvious protests, and I spent the following week on my couch. While in the hospital, my fever had come down, and I was hydrated again, so I knew I would be fine. I took digestive enzymes and put myself on a bland, mostly liquid diet, drinking only mineral water and eating only fruit smoothies and organic rice. I had stopped vomiting, and, gradually, my temperature decreased to 98.7°F. Thankfully, I had returned to "normal" by about a week later.

Once I was back on my feet, I knew I had to find a solution quickly or I would become ill again and eventually lose my intestines. I immediately purchased a copy of *Patient Heal Thyself*, and, at the risk of sounding clichéd, it changed my life. On its advice, I hastily changed my atrocious college-student diet radically from fast food and Rice-a-Roni to organic whole foods, such as fresh fruits and veggies. I also began taking dietary supplements—mainly probiotics, enzymes, and whole-food anti-inflammatories—while incorporating exercise, positive affirmations, and stress-management techniques into my life. I steadily improved, but despite all my efforts, something continued to trigger my symptoms.

At that point, I was not interested in merely getting myself better. Somehow, I felt compelled to help others going through this illness. Since being diagnosed, I had lost two friends to Crohn's disease. Experiencing their loss shook me awake to my calling. I knew what I was up against personally, but I also knew that knowledge is power. I needed to understand this disease from every angle possible. I decided to enroll in nutrition school, as my thirst for discovering the root causes of my illness had become unquenchable. I spent most of my free time with my nose in research books, medical journals, cookbooks, and the like. I found myself determined to uncover the answers that the medical community had lacked.

I talked to everyone and anyone who would listen about my condition. Later, at the suggestion of a classmate, I underwent genetic testing and discovered that I possess two copies of a gene (HLA-DQ) that predisposes me to severe gluten intolerance. Gluten is the protein found in wheat, rye, oats, and barley. And so, in the end, bread and pasta almost killed this lasagna-loving Italian girl. Go figure. I went on a gluten-free diet, and my digestion improved drastically: no stomach pain, no vomiting, no severe weight loss, and my acne, anxiety, depression, eczema, bloating, headaches, fatigue, and brain fog had disappeared. At age twenty-four, I finally felt "normal" for the first time in my life! Imagine that: After more than two decades, I *finally* knew the root cause of my mysterious stomach pains, aches, and noises. No words could describe the feeling. I felt as though I had finally arrived at the doorway to health.

My Approach

The standard medical treatment for IBD is typically surgery, bowel rest (food is delivered intravenously versus orally), and/or medications, with the goal of going into and remaining in remission. In my case, traditional methods didn't produce positive results. A holistic approach is much different, focusing on individual lifestyle, diet, relationships, exercise, spirituality, genetics, blood typing, and ancestry. Because no two people are alike, no treatments are exactly the same. This is the predominant theory upon which I have based the IBD principles featured in this book.

My approach to IBD incorporates close examination of the areas in your life and assessing the ways each aspect may contribute to, or exacerbate, your disease. I also place a heavy emphasis on evaluating vitamin, mineral, and amino-acid deficiencies. You will learn how a lack of these essential macronutrients can wreak havoc on your digestion, as well as your overall health and well-being. I will teach you how to discover and correct these imbalances with diet modification and supplement recommendations.

In relation to dietary changes for IBD, the main area of focus in my unique protocol consists of evaluating the presence of food *intolerances* versus food *allergies*. I have found the number of people with food intolerances to be far greater than the number of those with traditional food allergies (for further information on this subject see page 41). Intolerances cause a different type of reaction than allergies, and later in this book I will discuss why these reactions are so important for you to uncover. Because my approach enables you to discover your own unique dietary aversions, you can heal the inflammation in the gut caused by these foods. You will also learn how pH imbalance, bad bacteria overgrowth, leaky gut syndrome, toxicity, and candida overgrowth can negatively impact your health and the ways these elements can contribute to the onset of or mimic the symptoms of IBD.

The IBD Healing Plan and Recipe Book contains the answers you need to help alleviate all of these conditions so that you can get back to what is most important—living your life!

My Mission

Every day, while enjoying the simplicity of being able to eat normally once again or working with clients, I'm reminded of how regaining my health has been a tremendous blessing. The road to wellness wasn't easy for me, but traveling down that avenue allowed me to learn how to really listen to my body. The power to harness my health on a more conscious level is one priceless gift that I received from my illness. It also gave me the extraordinary passion I have for my mission: to help those with IBD embrace dietary and lifestyle changes so that they can live healthier and happier lives. In my opinion, too many people are suffering needlessly from IBD.

I have one wish for you: to get you off the IBD roller coaster for good. I want nothing more for you than for you to have your life back. I am living, walking, breathing, digesting proof that you *can* ditch this disease and live your days symptom free. Are you ready?

Note: The client stories in this book are based on true stories. However, the names have been changed to protect the identity of the clients portrayed.

Chapter 1

· · · · · · · · · · · · · · ·

Inflammatory Bowel
Disease 101

As you know from my life story and perhaps from your own experience, inflammatory bowel disease (IBD) is not something to take lightly. My clients and I share a common bond. We are a group of people who have learned to spot bathrooms a mile away, who must be very mindful of what we eat, and who have survived some of the nastiest belly pains ever. We have a relationship that only another person who has lived with IBD really understands. It is hard for someone who doesn't have IBD to fully grasp the physical pain and emotional upheaval that goes along with the condition. I find humor is one of the best tools for coping with the emotional side, because some of the stuff we deal with is a lot easier to manage if you can find a way to laugh through it. Most people cannot fathom going to the bathroom twenty times a day, farting in the middle of a dinner meeting, worrying about vomiting all over their professor's loafers, or wearing a diaper at the airport for fear they will have an accident midflight. If you have lived through situations like these, you're a champ. And in my eyes you're even cooler if you have found a creative way to handle or laugh at them.

One of my clients sure found a way to make himself laugh! It's no secret in the IBD world that going to the bathroom too frequently can cause pain—and soft toilet paper is welcomed! Here is a letter my client wrote to a major toilet paper manufacturer, a letter that still makes many people in my practice laugh!

Hello. My apologies for not having the Department/Manufacturing code; I hope this will find its way to the appropriate party. My fiftieth birthday celebration takes places this year. While I normally do not talk about my bathroom activities, I feel it may be appropriate with the maker of bathroom hygiene products.

I have been using fresh flushable wipes for the last three to four years, and I cannot go to the bathroom without them. If I forget them at home and am at work, I have to run out to the store to get them before I can use the restroom.

How can you resist the fresh feeling that they provide after your bathroom visits?

At this point, it has become quite comical to my wife, and as we were discussing things to put into my birthday party gift bags, I thought it might be fun to include fresh flushable wipes. While the cost of fresh flushable wipes is extremely reasonable, I was wondering if you would be willing to donate 150 packs to my birthday celebration? Think of it as a birthday gift to your biggest fan of flushable fresh wipes.

Either way, thanks for making a great product. While one would not normally describe one's toilet paper as life changing, your fresh flushable wipes really are.

Very truly yours,

Steven

Steven took his not-so-great bathroom situation and not only found relief with his beloved flushable wipes, but he also found the humor in his current state of affairs. I invite you to do the same.

If you have IBD, you will probably be able to relate to the stories of my clients in this book. Hopefully you can take solace in the knowledge that these wonderful people have been on a similar challenging path but are now thriving. Remember, you are not alone in your IBD journey.

Stephanie's Story

In my private practice, I am privileged to work with lovely and caring people. Because my experience with Crohn's is so intimate, it is no coincidence that working with IBD clients is always my favorite task. Working with Stephanie was no different.

I loved having sessions with Stephanie. She was quiet and studious, but she had a lot of courage under her soft exterior. She showed her bravery by waging a full-on battle to get her health back.

When Stephanie first came to see me, she had been suffering from Crohn's disease for a few years and was not doing any better than when she had first been diagnosed. The results of her colonoscopy were pretty severe: She had a significant amount of inflammation and about one dozen polyps. She had the noncancerous growths removed, but I feared that she had a long road ahead of her.

The day-to-day hustle and bustle of life proved to be too much for her illness-ravaged body. Stephanie experienced terrible malabsorption because of her distressed intestines and was malnourished as a result. Food was not appealing, so she lived on whole-wheat bagels and cereal. This client had days when she was too weak to get around, which proved especially devastating to her. She had nearly no support system at home, as her relationship with her husband was terribly strained. In fact, I suspected some verbal abuse, and occasionally Stephanie would tell me that she spent her time at home in fear.

The traditional treatment protocol for IBD usually starts with medication. The holistic nutrition approach is much different and involves examining the entire person being treated. In Stephanie's case, after I conducted an extensive health history, I suspected that her symptoms were related to a few environmental and lifestyle factors.

As part of our work together, I asked Stephanie a series of questions. First, I asked her to write about what her life would be like if she were well and had no health limitations. I told her to write as long as she liked and to be as realistic as possible. Then I asked her to put down what she thought was preventing her from getting well and what she thought might help. Finally, I asked Stephanie to map out what her life would look like in ten years.

It took her some time to finish, but eventually she produced this:

Limitations:
If I could rid myself of this damned disease, I would fly across the country and visit my sister, who I have not seen in a very

long time. I would be able to ride the train to work without worrying about finding a bathroom every ten minutes or being late because I spent too long in a bathroom! I would be free to do what I want to do, and I would no longer allow my disease to hold me back. I wouldn't miss social gatherings or work functions because of flare-ups. There are days where I simply avoid going out because I don't want to deal with the hassle. I just want my life back and I want the unbearable episodes of pain to stop.

What prevents me from getting well:
I know that I do not eat correctly, but some days, I just can't help myself. I enjoy eating cookies, and I really can't do without them. Why do I crave these foods so badly? I am also not hungry much of the time, and I am afraid of food because I am not really sure if what I am eating is setting off my stomach! I am sad much of the time, because I am lonely and feel sick. I don't have any support at home, because my husband does not help me. I think if I had more support, I would and could get well.

My life in ten years:
I would eat really well, as if it were second nature, and not struggle so much to eat healthy. I would be well, completely, and off medications. I would have more support in my life. I would be going out with my friends more and visiting my sister out of town more often, and I would be promoted from my current job position.

After going over each of her points, I showed Stephanie why a holistic approach would work for her. The root of some of her flare-ups seemed to be stress. She reported having more symptoms when at home than when she was with friends or other family members. She also knew that some foods affected her negatively but was not sure which ones. And she lacked energy, of course, because she was malnourished.

I tested the patient for food intolerances and found that she could not have wheat or dairy. Stephanie had several vitamin and mineral deficiencies, so I put her on supplements and tailored her elimination diet to address her sensitivities and deficiencies. She began a regime of digestive enzymes to assist with breaking down food, along with probiotics to rebuild the lining of her intestines and flush out bad bacteria. I also recommended that Stephanie begin an anti-stress/relaxation CD program from Lucinda Basset at the Midwest Center for Stress and asked her to arrange for bi-weekly outings with her girlfriends. I also advised her to get more sleep and to spend some time doing gentle exercise, such as yoga.

We worked together for six months, and Stephanie followed my recommendations and steadily improved. She got so much better that one sunny winter afternoon she came running into my office and announced, "Christie! I just wanted to report some good news to you! I had to have a colonoscopy before my appendix surgery to see if there would be any problems for the surgeon. The results were completely normal. No signs of inflammation. No signs of colitis or Crohn's activity!" The smile plastered on her face was priceless as she wrapped her arms around me. For Stephanie, many factors in her life ultimately "set off" her illness. Once she was able to find balance, she thrived and eventually was able to get off medication for good.

Important note: Keep in mind that you should never go off medication without speaking with your doctor first. My first concern is your safety!

The IBD Family

Crohn's disease, colitis, diverticulitis, ulcers, gastroesophageal reflux disease (GERD), hiatal hernias, celiac disease, irritable bowel syndrome (IBS)…the list of things that can go wrong in the digestive tract, esophagus, intestines, and stomach is overwhelming. *The IBD Healing Plan and Recipe Book* focuses on holistic treatment for Crohn's disease, colitis, and celiac disease. Throughout the text, markers indicate which recommendations apply to which diseases.

Readers with celiac disease should bear in mind that because the illness stems from genetic and dietary factors, the only treatment at this time is nutritional. You will greatly benefit from the gluten-free recipes in this book. If you have concurrent food sensitivities, you should also find this book helpful because most of the recipes don't contain the eight most common allergens. For those who have suffered for years with undiagnosed celiac disease, the vitamin and mineral assessments are helpful, as is the section on repairing your gut.

Readers with Crohn's and colitis should check out all the activities, quizzes, recipes, and recommendations, because everything in this book is tailored to your unique digestive issues.

Readers with IBS can still utilize the information in this book, even though IBS is considered a functional, less-severe illness that does not cause the same inflammation or damage that IBD does. Because most IBS symptoms and causative factors are similar in nature to IBD, you can fully take advantage of all the information and recipes this book offers. If a recommendation is specific to one condition, it is noted accordingly. Readers with diverticulitis or diverticulosis will find the recipes appealing, because most of them are free of nuts.

According to the Centers for Disease Control and Prevention (CDC), IBD is a broad category that describes conditions with recurring or chronic immune response and inflammation of the gastrointestinal tract. The two most common inflammatory bowel diseases are ulcerative colitis and Crohn's disease.

Here is a brief overview of the three diseases that exemplify the IBD family, including their associated symptoms.

Crohn's disease: This inflammatory condition typically manifests in the small intestine, causing diarrhea, vomiting, skin rashes, bowel obstructions, low-grade fever, chills, sweats, anemia, dehydration, and pain, in some cases severe. Without proper symptom management, a majority of those with Crohn's will eventually have surgery to remove all or part of the intestine. According to the *World Journal of Gastroenterology*, although advances in the medical management of Crohn's disease have decreased the need for surgery, it is estimated that between 70 and 90 percent of Crohn's patients will need surgical intervention at some point.[1] Recurrence rates following resection (surgery) remain high, and although not all symptomatic recurrences require surgery, it has been reported that surgical reintervention occurs in 25 to 35 percent of patients after five years and 40 to 70 percent after fifteen years.[2]

Colitis: This inflammatory condition generally affects the large intestine. Symptoms can be similar to Crohn's disease; however, pain is less common. Fatigue plays a large role with this illness due to additional malabsorption and nutrient loss. Colitis symptoms include constipation, diarrhea, skin rashes, bowel obstructions, high fever, and anemia.

Celiac disease: This disease is caused by the body's inability to digest the protein gluten or gliadin. Gliadin is a subset of gluten proteins and is also known as glycoprotein. Gluten and gliadin are found in wheat, rye, barley, oats, semolina, and durum flour, among other foods. Consumption of gluten for those who have celiac can lead to extensive damage of the villi, the white, fingerlike projections that live on the intestines and are responsible for nutrient absorption. Chronic inflammation caused by gluten consumption can cause the villi to flatten and lead to nutrient malabsorption. Symptoms of celiac include vomiting, diarrhea, constipation, gas, pain, bloating, fever, obstructions, vitamin and mineral deficiencies, and headaches.

Who Gets IBD?

According to the National Digestive Diseases Information Clearing House (NDDIC), in the United States, approximately 359,000 people were affected by Crohn's disease in 1998.[3] The NDDIC also reported the prevalence of ulceritive colitis to be about 619,000, meaning that approximately 1 million Americans suffered with IBD.[4] Generally, the onset of IBD occurs between ages fifteen to thirty. The Crohn's and Colitis Foundation of America suggests that hormone activity and puberty play a role in this illness, as do genetics and ancestry.[5]

Italian research published by the U.S. National Library of Medicine reveals people who are of European descent—primarily from Italy—seem to have a higher incidence of celiac disease than the rest of the world.[6] Because of the increase in individuals who are sensitive to gluten, Italian hospitals now screen babies for celiac disease at birth. Italian bakeries are even beginning to modify their bread recipes to include rice flour instead of traditional semolina to accommodate the growing celiac and gluten-intolerant population. European Jews also seem to have a higher incidence of IBD. The incidence of Crohn's disease and ulcerative colitis among white individuals throughout the world is approximately four times that of other races, with the highest rates reported to be in Jewish populations. The prevalence of Crohn's disease among the American Jewish population is approximately four to five times higher than in the general population. However, data suggest that the incidence rates in non-Jewish, black, and Hispanic populations are increasing.[7]

In an interview in the *Journal of Clinical Gastroenterology*, Dr. Charles Bernstein suggests that people who live in developed countries are more likely to be diagnosed with Crohn's or colitis as opposed to people who live in more rural areas.[8] From a nutritional standpoint, this trait is undoubtedly due to the overconsumption of processed, denatured foods that we are increasingly exposed to in industrialized nations across the world. I talk more about nutrition and how it relates to IBD in Chapters 2, 3, and 4.

According to the CDC, ulcerative colitis is more prevalent among ex-smokers and nonsmokers, whereas Crohn's disease is more prevalent among smokers.[9] A study by the *New England Journal of Medicine* found that seventeen of thirty-five colitis patients who were given 15 mg of nicotine daily actually showed improvement of symptoms over a short time period.[10] Bizarrely enough, no one is sure why nicotine seems to have a positive effect on patients with colitis and a negative effect on those with Crohn's, but the studies' results were consistent with epidemiologic findings that ulcerative colitis is a disease of nonsmokers and those who have recently stopped smoking.

The Science Behind IBD

Western science is unsure what causes Crohn's or ulcerative colitis, although it has developed a number of theories. The U.S. Department of Health and Human Services reports that those suffering from IBD have abnormal immune systems that can "attack" themselves. In a patient with Crohn's or colitis, the immune system appears to fight off bacteria that naturally occur in the digestive tract.[11] When the immune system reacts in this way, chemicals called cytokines are produced, causing the intestines to become inflamed. Once the intestines become inflamed, people begin to experience the symptoms of IBD, such as diarrhea and vomiting.

Western medicine does not support the theory that specific foods have a significant impact on digestive disease, which contradicts the theories of Eastern medicine. Eastern medicine dictates that nutrition, genetics, environment, stress, and microbial infections (bacterial or fungal in nature) are the paramount causes of digestive weakness. If the body is left in a state of microbial invasion, chronic stress, or poor nutritional balance over a long period of time, these weaknesses can become IBD (although this is not necessarily true of celiac disease, which is purely genetic in its onset). No one is really certain as to what triggers the gene for celiac disease to "turn on," although a common theory blames environmental factors, or epigenetics (see sidebar).

The University of Utah defines **epigenetics** as follows: The development and maintenance of an organism is orchestrated by a set of chemical reactions that switch parts of the genome off and on at strategic times and locations. Epigenetics is the study of these reactions and the factors that influence them.[12] In other words, our environment and lifestyle have a great deal to do with how our genes express themselves. If your great grandma died of cancer, you may say it's "in your genes." But what dicates if the gene actually turns *on*, and you wind up with cancer, or if it remains *off*? Your environment. Genes can change and develop into any disease if you live in a polluted area, consume a poor diet, eat foods that are contaminated with pesticides, don't exercise, and don't have a healthy life balance.

Common Treatment Methods Used in Western Medicine

Once you are diagnosed with IBD, you have many treatment options to consider and decisions to make. Whether you are a new IBD patient or a veteran to the disease, it is always wise to research your treatment options *before* committing to one. Of course, this is not always possible. For example, if you find yourself in an emergency setting, you are certainly not going to be running into the hospital with a stack of research books, nor will you have time to investigate surgery if you're in a life or death situation. However, most surgical procedures for Crohn's or colitis are elective and not conducted on an emergency basis, so most of the time, you will have the ability to discuss options with your doctor. Keep your relationship with your medical practitioner open so that they can answer any questions you may have regarding treatments. This section outlines the typical choices from Western medicine for treating Crohn's, celiac disease, and colitis.

Medications

Medications for Crohn's and colitis vary depending on the severity of your symptoms. Your doctor may prescribe antibiotics, laxatives, corticosteroids, pain medications, aminosalicylates, immunomodulators, or biological immune-suppressant treatments, such as infliximab. This option usually is not applicable for those with celiac disease, unless there is infection or inflammation from gluten ingestion present.

Surgery

For *Crohn's disease* the types of surgeries you may encounter are bowel resections, full removal of the large intestine, and/or strictureplasty (a surgery that removes accumulations of scar tissue, something fairly common in Crohn's patients). About 75 percent of Crohn's patients need surgery at some point to resolve issues such as fistulas, intestinal bleeding, or strictures in the bowel (constricted areas caused by scarring).[13]

For *colitis* patients the odds are a bit more favorable, with only 25 to 40 percent of individuals requiring surgical intervention.[14] Two types of surgery are most common, both involving the large intestine.

The first type of surgery is proctocolectomy with ileostomy. For many years, proctocolectomy has been performed along with a procedure called ileostomy. The ileum is the lowest part of the small intestine, and the word stoma means opening. An ileostomy—performed after the colon, rectum, and anus have been removed—involves bringing the end of the small intestine (ileum) through a hole (stoma) in the abdominal wall, allowing drainage of intestinal waste out of the body.

After the procedure, an external bag must be worn over the opening at all times to collect waste. The bag is emptied several times a day. The usual site for an ileostomy is the right lower abdomen just below the belt line, to the right of the navel. (For more information on ostomies, I recommend Dr. Craig A. White's *Positive Options for Living with Your Ostomy*.)

The second type of surgery that can be utilized with colitis is called a restorative proctocolectomy. This newer procedure, also called an ileoanal pouch anal anastomosis (IPAA), allows the patient to continue to pass stool through the anus. This procedure has become the most commonly performed surgical procedure for ulcerative colitis and is the preferred option for many people.

Psychological Intervention

Symptoms of digestive illness and anxiety often go hand in hand. Chronic illness and pain lower your tolerance for stress and can really take an emotional toll. Some patients are referred for counseling to cope with their condition.

Why a Holistic Approach?

Holistic wellness supports all systems of the body. Through my work with clients and my own personal experience, I have found that a well-rounded integration of individualized therapies for the patient serves as the best approach to improving IBD. When I studied at the Institute for Integrative Nutrition, we learned that the term "health" encompasses more than simply putting the right fuel into your body.

To maintain good health, you must not only change your overall diet but your overall *lifestyle*. A true holistic approach incorporates all areas of life into the makeup of your overall health. From here on out, I call these areas Primary Health Puzzle Pieces (PHPPs). While reading *The IBD Healing Plan and Recipe Book*, you will have the opportunity to implement lifestyle changes, permitting you to ameliorate these pieces of your health. I also focus on how the PHPP can impact your IBD and even exacerbate it! You will see that it is vital to adopt positive coping skills and techniques to avoid flare-ups. Treating IBD is not just about nutrition—your lifestyle matters, too!

The PHPPs that form your own unique health puzzle include:

- career
- creativity
- education
- exercise
- finances
- happiness

- home cooking
- home environment
- nutrition
- relationships
- social life
- spirituality

Working on Your Primary Health Puzzle Pieces to Manage IBD

Let's talk about determining which of your own PHPPs need some fine tuning. I recommend checking out the Wheel of Digestive Health exercise on page 35. Once you have completed this exercise, refer to the PHPP list above. Do any particular areas from the list or the Wheel of Digestive Health stand out for you? Focus on aspects that you suspect have an impact on your IBD first, and then go from there. For example, if you notice that you are stressed at work and that each day on your way to your job you feel ill, how does this contribute to your IBD? Is a situation with a coworker setting you off? Can you change jobs? Are you fearful of having a flare-up at work? Or if you notice a certain food has been triggering your symptoms, have you tried eliminating that food from your diet? Asking yourself these types of questions while completing the exercise *What Are Your Top Three Health Goals?* on page 33 will help you develop a plan for each area. You will be amazed at how you will innately know what is or isn't working for you. Having your goals mapped out will help hold you accountable and allow for an easy, practical approach to changing your lifestyle.

The primary areas that make up our lives, as listed above, are the "fruits of life" that truly nourish us on a spiritual level. As adults, we tend to forget about the importance of play, and we tend to forget about the things that makes us feel passionate about life. If this has happened to you, think about how this mind-set affects your IBD. We are spiritual beings living in a materialistic world. Because of the health emergency modern life has caused us, many of us are now re-evaluating our lives to determine what is truly important.

I believe happiness plays a large role in health and is certainly pivotal in PHPP management. It is not simply the act of eating healthy foods that contributes to your longevity and vitality—more importantly, it is what your life is like in each of the primary areas discussed above. Have you ever heard the phrase "laughter is the best medicine"? Research has shown that the simple act of smiling allows the body to release feel-good hormones, such as endorphins, which promote happiness and wellness. Think about a time when you were passionately in love, or when you were a child busy playing with friends but were called away for dinner. You could not have cared less about eating, because you were so involved with your lover or with play. Eating became secondary to living your life.

So although nutrition is paramount, it can be secondary to what is really important in life. However, it is essential to acknowledge what makes up your overall diet. Remember the old adage: You are what you eat. Being more conscious of the fuel you put into your body is a marvelous first step in determining how to improve your overall nutritional health. It is very important to understand how to achieve your own unique balance while looking at your PHPPs and to find the appropriate food intake that suits your specific digestive system.

The American Lifestyle and a Holistic Approach to Disease

Due to our unbalanced and busy lifestyle, many Americans are more sedentary than ever. Does this describe you? For instance, the average American only takes about five thousand steps per day,[15] or half of what's needed daily, according to Dr. Catrine Tudor-Locke's article regarding appropriate amounts of exercise; thus, we are certainly not moving around enough.[16] Many people eat out and on the run due to crowded schedules and poor planning. These choices add up after a while, and IBD patients should seriously consider their impact.

Since your IBD diagnosis, have you ever wondered whether the modern American lifestyle contributes to your illness? In Chapter 3 I include an in-depth explanation of the American diet, but right now, just look at your own lifestyle and see if you can pinpoint anything that triggers your IBD. Because a holistic approach to IBD includes ensuring a healthy balance between work and play, along with stress management, this is a valid point to examine.

Because I have witnessed such positive results from using a holistic approach, I am intrigued by any information on the connection between emotions and IBD. If you're interested in exploring this topic further, I recommend Dr. Peter Levine's book *In an Unspoken Voice: How the Body Releases Trauma and Restores Goodness*. It offers convincing biological explanations for the correlations between digestive problems and stress, and gastric motility and the nervous system.[17]

Dr. Levine also writes about Charles Darwin, who was interested in digestion (many believe that Darwin may have had Crohn's[18]). Darwin hypothesized that a strong connection exists between the heart and the brain, and that the two affect each other when it comes to illness. In Darwin's book *The Expression of the Emotions in Man and Animals* he cites the work of Claude Bernard, who speculated "that when the heart is affected it reacts on the brain, and the state of the brain reacts through the pneumo-gastric nerve on the heart; so that under any excitement there will be much mutual action and reaction between these, the two most important organs in the body."[19]

These ideas make a great deal of sense to me. The lining of the gut houses many nerves that govern sensory and motor functions to keep the digestive organs operating properly. Have you ever heard the phrase "nervous stomach"? It is not just a figure of speech—from an anatomical standpoint, it is a reality. Besides being intimately connected with the central nervous system, the digestive system is endowed with its own, local nervous system, dubbed the enteric, or second, nervous system. I love telling clients this. It really gives meaning to popular phrases like "I had a gut feeling about that" and "I have butterflies in my stomach."

It also explains why having a digestive disease can affect our moods tremendously. I routinely test my IBD clients' neurotransmitter levels. Neurotransmitters are responsible for producing certain hormones in the body, including serotonin, norepinephrine, and epinephrine (adrenalin). Many people are unaware that 95 percent of the body's serotonin (a hormone that helps us to feel good) is actually produced in the gut, not in the brain! When neurotransmitters are out of balance—for example, due to poor nutrition, such as inadequate levels of the amino acids tryptophan and tyrosine—we can become depressed. Therefore, maintaining a healthy digestive tract is important to keeping us feeling happy and healthy.

The problem is that most people with IBD do not absorb nutrients correctly, which puts us at a greater risk of neurotransmitter imbalance and also affects the production of adenosine triphosphate (ATP). ATP is a coenzyme used by the body to store and carry energy in the cells; it is the immediate energy source for most cellular activity. As such, it is intimately involved in all of our bodily processes.

As you can see, issues with nutrient absorption can lead to all kinds of problems—not just in the digestive system, but also in the nervous system, musculoskeletal system, immune system, and endo crine (hormone-production) system.

Still not convinced that lifestyle, nutrition, and IBD go hand in hand? Consider the following: In Michael Moore's documentary *Sicko*, Moore interviews people from France about health care, career, lifestyle, and how each element affects health. In the interview, Moore brings up the fact that the average American works forty to fifty hours weekly. This concept causes the French to laugh jovially. One gentleman stifles his laughter and comments, "Here in Europe, we only work thirty-five hours per week. We need to make time for what's really important in life—family. The Americans are so silly, running around like crazy. Your people work too much, and they are all of poor health! See what your working habits are doing to your country?"

The French credit their vitality to superior *free* health care, working less, and proper nutrition. Another woman who is interviewed brings up another interesting point: She claims the average person in France spends more money on high-quality, organic food and less on housing, thus explaining why their living arrangements tend to be more modest compared to those of Americans. It turns out, there is something to the more-holistic, balanced lifestyle French citizens experience.

In a first-of-its-kind study, the World Health Organization (WHO) has analyzed health-care systems around the world. Using five performance indicators to measure health-care systems in 191 member states, it finds that France provides the best overall health care, followed by Italy, Spain, Oman, Austria, and Japan. The WHO also claims that the health-care system in America costs a higher portion of its gross domestic product than in any other country but ranks 37 out of 191 countries in performance.[20]

Countries Ranked in Order of Longest Life Expectancy

1. France	21. Belgium
2. Italy	22. Colombia
3. San Marino	23. Sweden
4. Andorra	24. Cyprus
5. Malta	25. Germany
6. Singapore	26. Saudi Arabia
7. Spain	27. United Arab Emirates
8. Oman	28. Israel
9. Austria	29. Morocco
10. Japan	30. Canada
11. Norway	31. Finland
12. Portugal	32. Australia
13. Monaco	33. Chile
14. Greece	34. Denmark
15. Iceland	35. Dominica
16. Luxembourg	36. Costa Rica
17. Netherlands	37. United States of America
18. United Kingdom	38. Slovenia
19. Ireland	39. Cuba
20. Switzerland	40. Brunei

(source: World Health Organization Study on Life Expectancy)

How Can Blue Zones Teach You about Holistic Health?

Why are the French number one on the list of countries with the highest life expectancies? It is a valid question that makes you wonder whether the U.S. approach to disease control and prevention is really working. We are spending more on health care per capita, yet we are not ranked very high in terms of life expectancy. Because the French suggest our lifestyle negatively impacts our health, I invite you to look at a quaint U.S. town that serves as a testiment to the benefits of practicing a holistic lifestyle.

On April 19, 2010, *The Oprah Winfrey Show* featured a segment from Dr. Mehmet Oz about places called "blue zones," exclusive areas in the world where people live longer, healthier lives. In most places, the prospect of living to age one hundred sounds like a mixed blessing: Although some would consider a life of longevity a joyous accomplishment, others may be concerned that advanced age is often synonymous with diminished health and mental function. But this isn't the case in the blue zones.

In four hot spots around the globe, people live to be at least one hundred in great numbers. But the accomplishment is not only about longevity—blue-zone residents are happy, healthy, and spunky. The population regularly exercises, cares for its gardens, and lives as active, participating members of the communities. These people also stress the significance of eating delicious food and even having sex.

To find out what they're doing right—and what we're doing wrong—Winfrey and Dr. Oz looked to Dan Buettner, a writer for *National Geographic* who spent seven years researching his book *The Blue Zones: Lessons for Living Longer from the People Who've Lived the Longest.*

Wondering where blue zones are scattered throughout the world? One is found about 120 miles off the coast of Italy, in Sardinia, which fits the findings of the WHO study. Another is nestled in the extremely remote Nicoya Peninsula in Costa Rica. Only one is found in the United States, in Loma Linda, California.

What is Loma Linda's secret to longevity? Is it the citizens' holistically oriented lifestyle? You be the judge. Most of the population of this small city belongs to a Christian church that believes in eating only fresh, healthy, unprocessed foods, such as fruits, vegetables, and whole grains. The community is completely vegan, meaning it does not eat any animal-sourced foods, not even milk, eggs, and honey. Drinking and smoking are prohibited as well. Such lifestyle beliefs as practicing thankfulness and mindfulness are also very important to the people of Loma Linda. They try not to focus on their problems but on helping each other and being happy.

One story was particularly impressive: Dr. Ellsworth Wareham was a ninety-four-year-old heart surgeon who was still practicing, in addition to spending up to ten hours each week exercising and gardening. He very much believed in a holistic lifestyle, adopting a healthy spiritual practice and a low-stress lifestyle. He also promoted living medication free whenever possible. Another Loma Linda citizen, Marge, was 104 years old, rode a bike seven miles per day, and volunteered for seven different organizations. She adopted a daily ritual of mindfulness and being thankful and attributed her long life to this positive mind-set. She stressed the importance of taking one day of rest per week and planning regular time outdoors, mostly nature hikes. Dr. Oz reported, "These are certainly reasons why a holistic approach is appropriate for longevity."[21]

In my early Crohn's days, while in the hospital, I once had a doctor tell me, "Crohn's disease is a lifestyle disease. You need to change your lifestyle." Because our country focuses on "sick" care rather than preventative care, I had no clue what he meant at the time. "Change what?" I thought. Loma Linda, California, is a fine example of what holistic health care looks like when it is practiced correctly. I highly recommend you search online for this *Oprah Winfrey Show* episode, as it is quite inspiring, especially if you are having a bad IBD day. Marge is a great example of how living a holistic lifestyle can help you live a longer and happier life. Although Marge and Dr. Wareham do not have IBD, there is certainly something to be said about the benefits of examining your PHPPs.

Band-Aid Syndrome

Across the world, many of us have become accustomed to fixing problems the quick way—especially when it comes to our health. Consequently, we tend to rely heavily on prescription drugs to cure our diseases. I have had the privilege of working alongside many caring and intelligent doctors who prescribe medication as a last resort and only when it is clearly needed. This approach has always made sense to me, and it is what I always advise my clients. If you need to take medication for IBD, do so. But you also need to be well informed and remember because the cause of Crohn's and colitis is unknown, the medication is treating the *symptoms* of the illness rather than the root cause. I call this phenomenon the Band-Aid approach, treating symptoms but not always the cause of the disease. Many times, medications are not the best option because they can cause undesirable side effects. My intention is for you to discover what triggers your IBD symptoms, if possible, and find ways to cope with the disease holistically instead of covering it up with drugs. In case this proves not to be possible and you MUST take medications, below I outline the medications commonly used for Crohn's and colitis along with their associated vitamin and mineral deficiencies. The idea is for you to be able to successfully treat your IBD with medication while at the same time counteracting or addressing any nutrition problems that may arise from taking these medications. I have had the opportunity to work with many patients (with their physicians' assistance) who have been able to completely stop taking medication, and I personally have been medication free since 2004. However, you should never attempt to quit taking prescribed drugs without first consulting your doctor.

Risks of Prescription Drugs

According to "Death by Medicine," the groundbreaking 2003 medical report for *Life Extension Magazine* by Drs. Gary Null, Carolyn Dean, Martin Feldman, Debora Rasio, and Dorothy Smith, 783,936 people in the United States die every year from conventional medical mistakes.[22] The fully referenced report shows that 2.2 million people per year have in-hospital, adverse reactions to prescribed drugs. The number of unnecessary antibiotics prescribed annually for viral infections is 20 million; antibiotics fight bad bacteria, not viral infections, deeming them useless in cases of viral infection.

In many cases, conventional medicine can be quite effective. If you chop your finger off, most likely someone can stitch it right back on. If you have an emergency situation with your IBD, visiting a hospital is paramount and can likely save your intestines and help you get over a flare-up. Diagnostic technologies and medical treatments advance on a daily basis, and wonderfully dedicated and amazing practitioners and researchers are working hard to find cures for diseases. Medications can save lives in many situations, but in some cases, they can be dangerous if used long term; for example, the Crohn's disease drug 6MP can cause elevated liver enzymes. Elevations in these enzymes can indicate damage to the liver, thus taking this drug for prolonged periods of time may cause undesirable changes to liver functioning and health. The long-term use of steroid treatment, such as prednisone for Crohn's or colitis, is also cautioned against by most doctors because staying on this medication can cause all kinds of issues, including long-term immune-system damage, osteoporosis, and cataracts.

The bottom line: If you need medication, follow your doctor's advice and take it. Just make sure that you are well informed regarding the potential risks. It is also a good idea to analyze the risk-to-benefit ratio. For example, a medication that makes you feel worse than before you started taking it is obviously not your best treatment option. Don't be afraid to talk with your doctor about side effects. Ultimately, my goal for you would be to be in remission and off medication, but understand that achieving this goal will take time (and in some cases may not be possible), so treat your case individually.

IBD Medications and Nutritional Deficiencies

Because medications can be hard for the body to break down and alter the body's natural functions, it is important to monitor the vitamins and minerals that can be depleted while you are taking IBD drugs.

The following list of medications for IBD and their nutritional side effects is meant to inform you about your choices for Crohn's and colitis treatment. Address any questions with your medical practitioner, and if you suspect that you have any nutritional deficiencies, take this book to a trusted nutrition specialist who can help you design an individualized supplement regime that is appropriate. Completing a metabolic profile (from the lab Metametrix, discussed in later chapters) will also help you determine your specific vitamin, mineral, and amino-acid needs. A nutrition professional can then customize a supplement regime based specifically on your unique needs. This approach lets you maximize your body's reactions to taking medication without compromising your nutritional health.

The following recommendations are based on the book *Side Effects Bible*, by Fredrick Vagnini.

Common Drugs for Crohn's/Colitis

DRUG: Pentasa   **ALTERNATE NAMES:** Mesalamine
PURPOSE: Pentasa is an anti-inflammatory used to treat IBD. It acts locally in the bowel instead of tracking down inflammation elsewhere in the body. It does not work for everyone, but it can bring relief from abdominal pain for some.
POSSIBLE SIDE EFFECTS: Headache, nausea, inflammation of the pancreas, back pain, and weakness
WHICH NUTRIENTS ARE ROBBED: Folic acid

DRUG: Flagyl   **ALTERNATE NAMES:** Metronidazole
PURPOSE: Flagyl is an antiprotozoal drug, which means that it is designed to treat diseases caused by single-celled organisms. It can be used for IBS infections, trichomoniasis, amebiasis, giardiasis, and so forth.
POSSIBLE SIDE EFFECTS: Dizziness and headaches
WHICH NUTRIENTS ARE ROBBED: Vitamin K, *Lactobacillus acidophilus*, and *Bifidobacterium bifidum*

DRUG: Cipro   **ALTERNATE NAMES:** Ciprofloxacin
PURPOSE: Well-known for treating those with anthrax, Cipro fights bacteria by interfering with their ability to synthesize their DNA. This prevents a bacterial army from growing. In addition to anthrax, Cipro is also used to treat cases of Crohn's or colitis in which bacteria are believed to be a factor.
POSSIBLE SIDE EFFECTS: Restlessness, headache, and kidney failure
WHICH NUTRIENTS ARE ROBBED: Biotin, vitamin B-12, Inositol, vitamin K, thiamin, zinc, riboflavin, niacin, vitamin B-6, *Bifidobacterium bifidum*, and *Lactobacillus acidophilus*

DRUG: Entocort   **ALTERNATE NAMES:** Budesonide
PURPOSE: This corticosteroid is used to suppress the inflammation seen in Crohn's disease, thereby reducing symptoms. Use of this drug leads to remission in at least half of those with mild to moderate Crohn's disease located in certain areas of the intestines.
POSSIBLE SIDE EFFECTS: Headaches, nausea, and respiratory infection
WHICH NUTRIENTS ARE ROBBED: Vitamin A, vitamin B-6, folic acid, vitamin C, vitamin D, vitamin K, calcium, magnesium, potassium, selenium, zinc, and melatonin

DRUG: Nexium   **ALTERNATE NAMES:** Esomeprazole
PURPOSE: Esomeprazole is used to treat erosive esophagitis, gastroesophageal reflux disease, and, in combination with other drugs, duodenal ulcers caused by the *H. pylori* bacteria. Although it doesn't keep the exit door (the door between the stomach and the esophagus that controls the release of hydrochloric acid) shut, it does reduce the production of stomach acid.
POSSIBLE SIDE EFFECTS: Headache, flatulence, allergic reactions, such as hives, anaphylaxis, and asthma
WHICH NUTRIENTS ARE ROBBED: Vitamin B-12, iron, and sodium

DRUG: Prednisone **ALTERNATE NAMES:** Glucocorticoids
PURPOSE: Prednisone is one of the glucocorticoids, a group of drugs used to treat diseases in which inflammation is a problem. It puts a damper on inflammation in several ways, including decreasing the amount of T cells, B cells, and other immune-system soldiers in the blood.
POSSIBLE SIDE EFFECTS: Insomnia, nervousness, indigestion, and increased appetite
WHICH NUTRIENTS ARE ROBBED: Vitamin A, vitamin B-6, folic acid, vitamin C, vitamin D, vitamin K, calcium, magnesium, potassium, selenium, and zinc

DRUG: Reglan   **ALTERNATE NAMES:** Metoclopramide
PURPOSE: This drug stimulates the body's ability to digest food and decreases nausea.
POSSIBLE SIDE EFFECTS: Weakness, drowsiness, and restlessness
WHICH NUTRIENTS ARE ROBBED: Riboflavin

How to Adopt a Holistic Lifestyle: Making Positive Changes

You know the saying "Rome wasn't built in a day"? The best way to make long-lasting, positive lifestyle changes is to take baby steps. Think of the children's fable "The Tortoise and the Hare": Slow and steady wins the race. Most of the time, drastic changes only lead to regression. If you can slowly and comfortably allow yourself to transition into a healthy way of life, you will gradually become more conscious of your body's own unique needs. This awareness is known as bio-individuality.

The first step to making changes is to consider two important factors. First, you may be afraid to make a change. A large part of the reason patients don't always make supportive lifestyle choices is simply because they are scared of change, especially when it comes to doing things that may cause discomfort, such as confronting sugar addiction or ending a bad relationship. Second, you could lack the motivation to embrace an indulgence in self-care. As Oprah Winfrey says, "Motivation comes from doing." Choose a place to start, and use the following exercises to help you eliminate your concerns. This process will allow you to place your action steps into a manageable plan to balance your lifestyle and deliver ultimate health and happiness.

Take a Stand—Change Your Digestion!

Take the quiz below to determine how your digestion is affecting you. Then complete the goal exercise to define some health and nutrition goals for yourself. Finally, check out the Wheel of Digestive Health on page 35 to determine which areas of your life are affected by your IBD.

Quiz Quiz: How Is Your Digestion Affecting You?

 There is no time better than the present to start looking at how your digestion affects you. Answer the following questions, and tally your score at the end. See the answer key for your results.

1. **You feel like…**
   A. you can practically eat anything and your stomach seems unaffected
   B. everything you eat sets off your symptoms
   C. you cannot determine which foods bother you and which do not

2. **You have an important meeting at work this morning. You…**
   A. skip breakfast for fear of having to use the bathroom during the meeting
   B. eat light and pray for the best
   C. don't worry about it, because you can eat anything you want and will be just fine

3. **On average, you have bowel movements…**
   A. once a day
   B. 2–4 times daily
   C. 5 or more times daily

4. On average, you have problems with nausea or vomiting…
   A. never   B. occasionally   C. frequently

5. Have you ever suffered from skin rashes such as eczema or acne?
   A. yes   B. no

6. Do you have strong, repeated cravings for the same types of foods, such as bread or dairy?
   A. never   B. occasionally   C. frequently

7. Do you suffer from frequent bouts of depression or anxiety?
   A. never   B. occasionally   C. frequently

8. Do you experience stomach cramping?
   A. never   B. occasionally   C. frequently

9. Do you have any other autoimmune problems, such as diabetes, cancer, fibromyalgia, or MS?
   A. yes
   B. no
   C. I don't know, as I've never been tested

10. Do you experience frequent infections and/or colds? (Example: Do you normally have a cold more than two times per year?)
    A. yes   B. no

11. Have you been on antibiotics more than three times in the past year?
    A. yes   B. no

12. Have you experienced any major loss in the past year or suffered a great deal of stress?
    A. yes   B. no

13. At mealtimes you…
    A. eat slowly
    B. inhale your food

14. At mealtimes you…
    A. read a magazine or watch TV
    B. sit undistracted or with others to eat

15. Do you feel that your digestion has affected your quality of living?
    A. no   B. somewhat   C. tremendously

Scoring Your Quiz

Here are the point levels for each answer. Tally them up and look at the information below to see how your digestion is affecting you.

QUESTION	ANSWER A	ANSWER B	ANSWER C
1	1	2	3
2	3	2	1
3	1	2	3
4	1	2	3
5	2	1	
6	1	2	3
7	1	2	3
8	1	2	3
9	2	1	
10	2	1	
11	2	1	
12	2	1	
13	1	2	
14	2	1	
15	1	2	3

My total score: _____

Score 15–20: Low Priority

Your digestion seems to bother you on occasion, perhaps when you are stressed or have just made poor food choices. Nonetheless, it is something you are concerned about and have possibly questioned. A great way to see how your digestion affects you is to keep a food diary, like the one featured in Chapter 2. This exercise will allow you to determine any food sensitivities. You should also complete the Wheel of Digestive Health exercise on page 35. Look at all of the aspects of the circle to see where you may be lacking. As the holistic perspective dictates, your digestive issues may not be entirely related to your food intake.

Evaluate the amount of time you are spending taking care of yourself, your relationships, and your stress levels. See if you can determine a factor that might be contributing to your IBD, and use the goals sheets in this chapter to devise a game plan for getting your life on the right track. Keep both a digestive and food diary to learn what triggers or improves your symptoms. I would start by jotting down the number of bowel movements you have per day and then marking the consistency (i.e., soft or well-formed). After tracking this activity, you may be able to see a pattern (for example, each time you have bread, your bowel movements may be loose, or you notice a change each time you are stressed). Keeping this journal for a couple of weeks can do wonders, allowing you to become more conscious of how your body reacts to diet and personal situations. If the idea of keeping a journal doesn't float your boat, lab testing can be preferable and yields accurate results. Chapter 2 offers more information about this process.

Consult your doctor to evaluate your symptoms as well.

Score 21–30: Medium Priority

If you are experiencing any of these symptoms, you should schedule a visit with your doctor. Based on the answers you provided, your IBD is really affecting your life. It may be causing you to avoid social situations as a result of the embarrassment that goes along with digestive illness. You may have resorted to over-the-counter products or are presently taking prescription medications to control your symptoms. Try following the supplement recommendations and the anti-inflammatory diet in this book. You should also contact one of the labs listed in the Resource section to be tested for food intolerance. You can try to identify food intolerance on your own by keeping a food diary and logging your bowel movements and digestive symptoms as suggested above. But because reactions to food can be delayed up to seventy-two hours, it may not always be possible to determine intolerances strictly by examining the journal. For this reason, lab testing is preferable and yields accurate results. Chapter 2 offers more information about this process.

You should also complete the Wheel of Digestive Health exercise on page 35 to determine whether an unbalanced lifestyle is contributing to your digestive issues. Once you have completed the circle, look at the goal sheets and design a plan for what you would like to work on first.

Score 31–39: High Priority

Based on the answers you provided, your digestion is a huge concern for you, to say the least. A good workup by your gastroenterologist is warranted at this point. Follow the supplement recommendations in this book and measure your intake of processed foods, sugar, cakes, and the like. Keep a food diary, get tested for food intolerance, evaluate your stress levels, and adhere to an anti-inflammatory diet. You should also consider following the recommendations for the low- and medium-priority scores as well. Read on to discover more ways to alleviate your symptoms. It is crucial to reach out for help before your health situation becomes out of control.

Worksheet: What Are Your Top Three Health Goals?

List your top three health goals. They can be anything from clearing up constipation to improving your diet to drinking more water.

Example:	I would like to eat healthier.
Goal #1:	
Goal #2:	
Goal #3:	

What Prevents You from Meeting Your Goals?

List one item for each goal, detailing the reasons you are currently prevented from achieving your goals.

Example:	I eat on the run, and I do not cook my own food. I rely on other people to prepare meals for me. I also like to eat a lot of sweets and drink coffee on a frequent basis.
Goal #1:	
Goal #2:	
Goal #3:	

What Can You Do Meet Your Goals?

Let's plan out some baby steps to help you meet your health goals. Talk them over with a trusted friend and ask them to hold you accountable. For each goal you designate, take consistent action toward reaching it. Keep this list on your refrigerator to make sure that you are clear on what you need to do to achieve optimum health. Good luck!

Example:	I can cook at home more often. I can eat healthier snacks if I prepare them from home. I can go food shopping once a week. I will also buy fresh-cut fruits, vegetables, nuts, and whole-grain pretzels instead of sugary snacks.
Goal #1:	
Goal #2:	
Goal #3:	

Food for Thought

When embarking on a quest to improve your digestive health, you should look at much more than what's on the surface. We tend to blame our health on elements that have nothing to do with why we are actually sick.

For example, if you can't stand your living situation and your spouse is constantly stressing you out, what negative impacts do you think it has on your digestive symptoms? Recall Stephanie, whose strained living arrangements and fear fueled negative digestive symptoms on most occasions. Many people do not realize that *their own environment can cause so much stress that it actually causes health problems.* Here is another example: I once had a friend who faced so much anxiety from his job that he wound up having a heart attack. It was his wake up call to take a step back and realize how his negative attitude involving his work had a great deal to do with his negative food choices. He had been eating unhealthily to bury his toxic emotions, which contributed greatly to his health calamity.

Perhaps another example is more fitting for you. Are you a workaholic, living without a healthy balance between work and play? How do you think leading a lifestyle of that nature can affect you? Review Stephanie's case. At the peak of her illness, she was suffering from a great deal of mental anguish due to a strained relationship with her verbally abusive husband. How do you think her relationship status affected her Crohn's disease? You get the point. You are not only what you eat but also what you think!

Worksheet: Wheel of Digestive Health

This worksheet is inspired by my school, the Institute for Integrative Nutrition, and is adapted from its version to suit the needs of an IBD patient.

The Wheel of Digestive Health (see Figure 1 below) incorporates all the factors from the earlier section titled "Why a Holistic Approach?" This unique wheel helps you clarify which of the areas of your life are balanced and which are in need of a tune-up. On a scale of 1 to 10, with 1 being very unhappy and 10 being ecstatic, rate how you feel about each area of your life. Pick one area per month to focus on. You can use the goal sheets on the previous two pages to plan action steps for anything that you would like to change in your Wheel of Digestive Health. Happy planning!

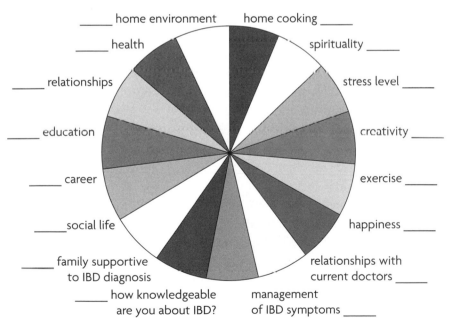

FIGURE 1. Wheel of Digestive Health

Chapter 2

Food Intolerance and Inflammatory Bowel Disease

Think you don't have any food intolerances? Think again, friend. You may be very surprised to find that you do! The same story applies to many of the clients I work with! They are usually shocked to see labwork coming back revealing that an unsuspecting food is causing their body harm!

Just like them, I was in disbelief when it came to food intolerance. When I was sick, I didn't really love food all that much, since it didn't seem to love me back. But on the rare occasion when I was hungry, all I could think of was bread. It seemed to "coat" and soothe my stomach. So for the longest time, I thought glutenous foods were "helpful" for my angry, old belly. As it turned out, we all know that gluten is my number one arch enemy.

This is where I really began to look at the role of food intolerance and IBD and how it affects people. In my first two years practicing, I came across a wealth of research to support the theory of food intolerance, and I really began to wonder what its role was in Crohn's disease. I knew from Jordan Rubin that food quaility was important and had that covered. In reading the *Specific Carbohydrate Diet* by Elaine Gottschall, I knew that her theory about avoiding grains made a great deal of sense, but wondered if it covered all the bases. I needed to learn more to fully understand what I was dealing with.

Early in 2009 I was still on my neverending quest for knowledge regarding diet and IBD when I met Dr. Robert Melillo. He was also on the same journey, learning about food intolerance, only he was studying its role in neurobehavioral disorders, like autism and

ADHD. Despite the differing reasons we were both on this path, learning from a brilliant professor and doctor served me well—and helped me to formulate this *IBD Healing Plan and Recipe Book*.

Frank's Story

Frank, a gentleman in his fifties, came into my private practice one day. He had suffered with Crohn's disease for close to thirty years. Initially, I was taken aback by this number because he had been suffering for an entire *decade* longer than myself! But I instantly connected with him, admiring Frank's ability to display such resilience. I respected his character for having been on such a long health journey that began with his diagnosis in the early 1980s when Crohn's disease treatments were very minimal at best. Even at the time of this writing, inflammatory bowel disease (IBD) is not fully understood, so you can imagine what he had been through. On the day of our first meeting, Frank was a gaunt 150 pounds standing nearly six feet tall and had a remarkably pale complexion. I could not help but gasp inwardly, knowing he was in a bit of trouble.

Frank's intake was interesting. He had somehow managed to avoid surgery over the past thirty years, but his doctor was really pushing for it at that point, as he was so grossly underweight for his build. Frank noticed that certain foods, such as dairy, triggered his symptoms. Ironically, copious amounts of ice cream, milk, and cheese were still quite prevalent in his diet, despite the fact that they seemed to cause cramping and vomiting episodes. It was strongly indicated that dairy was the main issue, and I suspected he was addicted to it. An addiction would surely account for why he chose to consume it, despite the obvious trouble it caused him. (I discuss more about food intolerance and addiction later in this chapter.) I tested him for bad bacteria overgrowth and oxidative damage along with food intolerances. Blood work revealed that Frank had severe intolerance to eggs and dairy and a significant amount of bad bacteria overgrowth in his intestines.

I recommended probiotics to help repopulate good bacteria and the amino acid glutathione to repair the lining of the intestinal walls. We worked diligently to eradicate dairy and eggs in his diet, and I educated him about some tasty, healthy milk alternatives, such as those made from hemp, almond, and rice. We also added some pancreatic enzymes, including bromelain, to control inflammation.

Lo and behold, I watched the real Frank reemerge right before my eyes. The glow came back to his cheeks, and, more importantly, the spark returned to his step. Frank's wife told me that Frank would usually become very depressed when his disease would act up. She knew he was beginning to feel better when he slowly started to emerge from the basement, which is where he felt most comfortable when he was ill. His appetite returned after many years of his being disinterested and disgusted by foods. After six months of bi-weekly nutrition counseling and monitoring, Frank weighed a healthy 190 pounds. Needless to say, we were both thrilled. Five years later and Frank still reports doing well, as long as he refrains from eating eggs and dairy and keeps his stress levels at bay.

Food Intolerance and IBD

At some point or another, you may have pinpointed certain foods that set off your digestive symptoms as Frank did. Perhaps your doctor recommended that you omit dairy, fried, or spicy ingredients from your diet to see how you feel. By trial and error, you may have even noticed that some foods aggravate your IBD. Have you ever observed that you stick with the same foods simply because they are "safe," meaning they don't seem to activate your IBD symptoms when you consume them?

As someone with IBD, you can develop a fear and an aversion to food over time. You might be scared of eating prior to a public outing due to the anticipatory anxiety around finding a restroom. Or perhaps you experienced a flare-up after eating and never wanted to ingest the associated food again. I once had a client with colitis who was triggered after drinking a popular weight-loss shake. Once she realized this beverage was causing her symptoms, she was disgusted by it and never drank it again. In fact, just *thinking* about the shake made her queasy. These are just a few reasons why identifying any food intolerances should be a priority. Knowing what you can and cannot consume will lessen your anxiety around eating. Over time, you will enjoy many foods again, because you will know that you can safely have them without provoking your illness. This chapter explores how food intolerances may affect you and your IBD.

Understanding Your Immune System

To understand the concept of food intolerance, you must first understand the unique immune responses of individuals with IBD, which differ from the responses of individuals who have normal, healthy digestion.

The immune system is the body's defense system against foreign invaders such as infectious organisms. It is made up of many different parts, because attacks can come in many forms. When the body is attacked, a series of "alarms" goes off, alerting the immune system as to what type of attack is occurring. The body then initiates a specific defensive action and counterattack. An antigen is a substance that causes the body to initiate this immune response. Think of antigens as enemy agents. Antigens can be foreign substances, such as bacteria, viruses, allergens, a parasite, or a transplanted organ. Antigens can also be produced by the body, such as toxins created by the body's cells. Once the enemy (antigen) is recognized, the body produces antibodies in response. Antibodies are specialized proteins manufactured by white blood cells that bind to, and thus neutralize, antigens. Think of antibodies as the body's defensive troops.

In Crohn's disease, colitis, and celiac disease, antigen production appears to be caused by a dysfunctional inflammatory response in the gastrointestinal tract. Inflammation is the body's natural attempt to heal by sending immune cells to the site of an injury or invader. Researchers hypothesize that this immune response in both ulcerative colitis and Crohn's disease may be triggered by bacteria or viruses, by material in the intestinal contents (such as products from food digestion or intestinal bile), or by a defective signal from the body's own cells, called an *autoimmune response*. Inflammation results in pain, heat, redness, and swelling of the tissue, known as *edema*. Chronic inflammation can impair the proper function of tissues and organs.

Antibodies, also called immunoglobulins, are divided into five classes, enabling them to recognize and fight a wide spectrum of antigens. The classes of antibodies are comparable to different branches of the military. Each branch has its own function and is responsible for a certain type of immune reaction. Here is a brief overview of the five types of immunoglobulin:

1. IgG—the most common immunoglobulin in the body (making up about 75 percent of all antibodies), and the body's main defense against bacteria and viruses. May also be involved in the production of inflammation-causing cytokines, triggered by reactions to certain foods.

2. IgM—involved in fighting blood infections and in triggering production of immunoglobulin G.

3. IgA—predominant in the mucous membranes of the respiratory and digestive tract and in saliva and tears; functions as the body's first line of defense against invading foreign substances. As the chief antibody in the membranes of the gastrointestinal and respiratory tracts, it is important for those with IBD. You may have had bloodwork done to check your IgA levels. If they are elevated, it means there is a disturbance in the mucosal lining of the intestines.

4. IgE—present primarily in the lungs, skin, and mucous membranes; most involved in the expulsion of intestinal parasites and in allergic reactions.

5. IgD—present in blood serum in small amounts, and the least understood of the antibodies.

Throughout the rest of this book, I will mostly discuss IgG and IgE reactions, as they can be associated with food and can therefore greatly impact IBD. IgA is also significant in those with Crohn's and colitis, since IgA is secreted from the mucosal tissue lining the intestines. At this time, there are no extensive testing panels for food-based IgA reactions; however, I suspect they will be developed and utilized in the future.

What Parts of the Body Does the Immune System Attack?

An immune system response can affect or "attack" four areas of the body, including:

1. the entire digestive tract, including the small and large intestines, colon, anus, and esophagus

2. the brain

3. the skin (Do you have skin conditions, such as eczema or psoriasis, acne, or rosacea?)

4. the respiratory tract (Do you have asthma, environmental allergies, ear infections, or tubes in your ears?)

If you notice that you have any of the above symptoms, such as skin issues or asthma, in addition to IBD, these health concerns are likely related to the way your immune system functions. You may find that as you are working on your diet, especially if you have food intolerance, avoiding reactive foods will help health issues other than IBD as well.

Environmental Factors That Can Affect the Immune System

A "threat or invader" to the body could be any environmental factor, including mold spores in your basement, a slice of cheese, toxins, bacteria, virus, and fungus. A normal immune system seeks out the threat and sends antibodies to attack. But because of the autoimmune attributes of IBD, the immune system begins to assault *their very own bodies*—specifically, the intestines—instead of the mold, cheese, or other irritant triggering the response.

IgE and IgG Food Allergies and Food Intolerance— What Is the Difference?

The primary difference between the two immune system reactions highlighted in this book is that allergic reactions are immediate and can be life threatening without prompt medical attention, while intolerance reactions are delayed. Therefore, exposure to elements that could trigger the latter can affect long-term overall health and well-being.

Food Allergies vs. Food Intolerances/Sensitivities

Food allergies and food sensitivities/intolerances are not the same! This reference chart highlights the most distinct details, so you can clearly see and understand the differences between the reactions.

▌Differences Between IgE Food Allergy and IgG Food Intolerance

IGE FOOD ALLERGY	IGG FOOD INTOLERANCE/SENSITIVITY
Immediate (within minutes) hypersensitivity response	Delayed hypersensitivity response (0–72 hours from initial exposure)
Usually a reaction to foods you eat infrequently	Usually a reaction to foods you eat frequently
Causes body to produce histamine	Causes body to produce inflammatory chemicals called cytokines, which cause inflammation in respiratory tract, gut, brain
Can be immediately life threatening, cause anaphylaxis	Can cause food addictions, "picky" eating
Generally affects airways	Associated more commonly with autoimmune disease

Immediate Hypersensitivity—IgE

Usually, if you have a true food allergy, you are made aware of it pretty early on in life. The majority of patients know if they have a food allergy because allergies produce immediate reactions in the body, such as hives, watery eyes, itching, sneezing, or, in the most severe case, life-threatening anaphylactic shock. Anaphylactic shock is a sudden, severe allergic reaction characterized by a sharp drop in blood pressure and breathing difficulties following a preliminary or sensitizing exposure to a foreign substance, such as a drug or food. The reaction may be fatal if emergency treatment, including epinephrine injections, is not given immediately. For example, if each time you have a strawberry you break out in hives or need an epi-pen to counteract the histamine reaction, you know you are dealing with a food allergy.

This immune-system response is called an IgE reaction, which is a true, bonafide allergy. Although some patients with Crohn's, colitis, or even celiac also have IgE food allergies, their presence does not seem to be as prevalent as IgG.

Delayed Hypersensitivity—IgG

Today, health practitioners are examining other environmental- or food-based reactions that can have negative impacts on health. This reaction is known as an IgG antibody reaction and it is the type of immune system response I focus on because of its prevalence in those with IBD. I have witnessed great improvement after eliminating IgG reactive foods from my own diet, and I have seen many other people benefit from doing the same. IgG reactions differ from a typical food allergy by *not* producing the quick reaction that someone with an allergy may experience. Although they are not immediately life-threatening, like their IgE counterparts, IgG reactions to food cause harm over time by stimulating the body to produce inflammatory chemicals called cytokines. Cytokines can affect the small and large intestine, wreaking havoc on the digestive system and leading to undesirable reactions, such as damage to various parts of the intestines. When the intestines become inflamed, the passageways begin to narrow and thicken, causing villi damage and malabsorption. All these symptoms contribute to IBD flare-ups. Cytokines can also be produced in the respiratory tract and brain, where they can cause problems such as difficulty breathing and difficulty concentrating—more potential (secondary) symptoms of digestion gone awry.

IgG sensitivities can be tricky to recognize, as they are delayed hypersensitivity reactions that may not show up for six to seventy-two hours. In other words, you can eat a piece of bread on Monday but not display a reaction until Wednesday. How would you know that the symptoms were caused by something you had ingested days ago? And therein lies the problem: Most people don't make the correlation. Most will argue that they would know whether a particular food triggers their IBD symptoms. In many cases, I have found that people are usually addicted to the very foods they are intolerant to. This is seen frequently in those with IBD who only feel comfortable sticking to a few "safe foods," such as bread and crackers.

Food Addiction, Leaky Gut
Syndrome, and IgG Reactions

How can you be addicted to a particular food? It all starts with the vicious cycle known as leaky gut syndrome. Researcher Dr. Robert Melillo believes this syndrome occurs because of a neurological component that involves immaturity in either of the two brain hemispheres. Most people are unaware of such developmental delays in their adult life and survive socially and academically. However, physical ramifications of this phenomenon, deemed by Melillo as "Functional Disconnection Syndrome," can actually cause leaky gut, because the nervous system is affected.[1]

When the brain is immature, the digestive system remains immature as well.

Two basic parts of the nervous system control regulation of the digestive system:

1. **the sympathetic nervous system:** Also known as the fight-or-flight system, this system is the basic survival system that everyone is born with. We come into the world screaming, kicking, and fighting to survive thanks to this portion of the nervous system. When we are born, we have very fast pulse rates and heartbeats; we breathe in a rapid, shallow way; we can't really digest solid food; and we don't sleep well. Our bodies are stressed out just by trying to survive.

2. **the parasympathetic nervous system:** As we grow and develop different and more mature functions, such as walking and talking, this other part of the nervous system activates. Also known as the rest-and-digest system, this system inhibits and quiets the flight-or-flight system. It slows the heart and pulse rates, allowing us to take deeper, slower breaths to take in more oxygen. It also slows down the digestive system and increases the flow of acid and blood that allow us to digest and to absorb nutrients from food.

If either side of the brain remains immature, the nervous system will always be stuck in fight-or-flight mode. This state causes a release of stress hormones that affect the whole body by making the individual's digestive system and body functions constantly "stressed out." This stress affects the digestive tract in three primary ways:

1. The body does not produce enough secretions, such as acid and digestive enzymes, to break down and digest food properly.

2. The digestive muscles may have weak muscle tone.

3. Poor circulation to the stomach and intestinal lining causes malabsorption.

All of the above conditions result in the loss of nutrients, minerals, and amino acids. They can also break down the stomach lining, a condition known as leaky gut.

When leaky gut is present, the lining of the intestines becomes very permeable, meaning food particles can easily leak into the bloodstream although they do not belong there. When a protein such as casein, the protein in dairy, is not completely digested, it remains in the body in a form called a polypeptide that can actually "leak through" the walls of the intestines and trigger an immune response.

Many of the polypeptides that form from undigested foods create opiate chemicals. When gluten or casein is consumed by a patient who is sensitive or intolerant, the opioid receptors are activated in the brain due to the formation of polypeptides, causing the body to produce a chemical called glutomorphin or casomorphin. Gluten is a protein found in wheat, rye, oats, and barley, while casein is the protein found in all dairy products. Most people consume these proteins routinely, as they make up a large portion of the standard American diet. As a result, you can actually crave the foods that you are most sensitive to, because they produce morphinelike effects on the body.

Recall Frank's case presented earlier. Even though he understood that dairy was affecting him negatively, he still ate it. Why? Because each time he ate dairy, although he was not consciously aware of it, he felt "high." Eating small amounts of these proteins caused his body to produce these morphinelike chemicals, which in turn made Frank have constant cravings for dairy.

Common Sensitivities

Someone with Crohn's or colitis may be sensitive to any food, but the most common sensitivities are to gluten and casein. These sensitivities are common because wheat and dairy were rare commodities until about ten thousand years ago. Although this seems to be a substantial amount of time, consider that for tens of thousands of years prior, grains were not part of the human diet. *The Blood Type Diet* by Dr. Peter D'Adamo claims the most common blood type, type O, originated as far back as 25,000 BC, when man consumed a diet consisting of animal protein, fruits, and vegetables. His theory is that the modern diet is therefore not suitable for people with type O blood, because grains were not consumed until many years later.[2] Approximately 80 percent of the average diet consists of wheat and gluten, but some humans have not evolved enough to have developed the appropriate digestive enzymes to assimilate these proteins. So for many with IBD, the hardest foods to digest actually make up the majority of their diet.

The Top Eight Allergens

The most common allergens (IgE reactions) humans contend with today are:

1. dairy
2. wheat
3. eggs
4. shellfish
5. tree nuts
6. soy
7. corn
8. peanuts

Although these foods are the most common allergens, they are also the most commonly experienced food intolerances.

Food Intolerance and Proteins

Notice that almost all the foods on the above list are proteins. Proteins can be a real problem for those with IBD. Why? Some people do not produce enough of an enzyme called protease, which breaks down proteins. Protein breakdown can also become an issue if there is a problem with the way the body utilizes amino acids.

Amino acids are the building blocks for protein. If you have micronutrient malabsorption due to villi damage from chronic inflammation in your intestines, you may have trouble breaking down proteins. Micronutrients are the nutrients that produce ATP (energy) in the cells, such as vitamins, minerals, fatty acids, and essential amino acids. When intestinal villi are damaged, your body cannot adequately absorb proper nutrition. As a result, you may stop producing the enzymes and amino acids necessary for proper digestion to occur. In a randomized study completed by the Division of Gastroenterology in Toronto, Canada, forty patients with Crohn's disease were given amino acids to determine whether they were an effective method of symptom control. The study showed that 84 percent of patients experienced remission after six months of amino-acid therapy coupled with a low-fat diet.[3]

Because many people with IBD have trouble breaking down specific proteins, it is necessary to find substitutes for these proteins. If testing determines that you are intolerant to one or more of the eight most common allergens, fear not: Many products available are great replacements—so great, in fact, that you probably won't even miss your offending foods.

Does this description of food intolerance strike a chord with you? Think very clearly about the dietary choices you make on a daily basis, and remember that each bite of food affects how you feel physically and mentally. Take the quiz below to determine whether you possibly suffer from IgG food intolerance.

Quiz Do You Have Food Intolerance?

☑ Score 2 points for each symptom that you experience more than three times per week. Tally your results and check out the answer key at the end. Follow up with your doctor if you are experiencing any of these symptoms, as they can indicate a flare-up or another serious health condition. Also note that having one or more of the symptoms below does not automatically mean they are caused by an aversion to food.

Digestive Symptoms—Do you suffer from:

☐ abdominal cramping   ☐ acid reflux
☐ abdominal pain   ☐ bloating after meals

☐ constipation/diarrhea
☐ difficulty gaining/losing weight
☐ excessive flatulence
☐ gallbladder abnormalities
   (i.e., difficulty digesting fats)
☐ hemorrhoids

☐ indigestion
☐ itchy anus
☐ mouth ulcers
☐ nausea/vomiting
☐ sinus congestion
☐ water retention

Total score = ___ /30 points

Nervous System Symptoms — Do you suffer from:

☐ addictions
☐ behavioral problems (such as
   hyperactivity/ADHD)
☐ brain fog (inability to think
   clearly that has progressively
   gotten worse)
☐ clumsiness
☐ constant hunger
☐ dark under-eye circles

☐ depression and/or anxiety
☐ food cravings
☐ headaches
☐ insomnia
☐ irritability
☐ memory loss
☐ migraines
☐ mood swings

Total Score: ___ /28

Total Score from Nervous System and Digestive System Sections: ___ /58

Score 0–16: Low Priority

Your symptoms could possibly be indicative of food intolerance, but it is less likely with a score this low. Perhaps you do not have food intolerance but are eating in a way that is unbalanced for your body. Notice the foods you are taking in. Are you eating too much protein? Maybe you are eating too little? Are you eating enough fruits and vegetables? Are you eating a lot of sugar? Have you recently switched IBD medications? All of these can aggravate IBD, so it is important for you to become conscious of your food choices.

To achieve a higher level of awareness, you'll want to keep a food diary like the one featured earlier in this chapter. After you have done this for several weeks, look for patterns to determine whether any specific food is setting off your IBD. If you find that one or more foods are bothering you, follow an elimination diet (see the instructions later in this chapter). This process will allow your body to heal from the inflammation caused by the food intolerance, and you should start to feel better.

If no food seems to be causing your symptoms, evaluate other factors. How is your stress level? What is going on with your Primary Health Puzzle Pieces (PHPPs, discussed in Chapter 1)? Check all the areas of your Wheel of Digestive Health (see page 35) to decide whether you can work on any particular area to improve your health. Last, but certainly not least, if you are experiencing any of these symptoms, make an appointment with your gastroenterologist.

Score 18–38: Medium Priority

With a score in this range, it is likely that you have a food intolerance. Schedule an appointment with your doctor to discuss the health concerns you checked off above. If your doctor rules out other causes as the source of your symptoms, your best bet is to do two things:

First, keep a food diary for a week or so. You may be able to immediately identify an offending food. Look for any symptoms that cause you discomfort, such as bloating, gas, or even moodiness or sadness for no particular reason.

If the food diary doesn't answer your questions, contact a health practitioner who does testing for IgG food intolerance. A nutritionist, chiropractor, or naturopath can usually order tests like this. You can also contact Metametrix Laboratories at (800) 221-4640 or http://www.mctametrix.com to order a Triad Profile, which uses blood and urine samples to test for up to ninety food intolerances and organic-acid profiles from which individualized vitamin/mineral/amino-acid formulas may be ordered. This test allows you to determine your food sensitivities accurately and even see which specific vitamin and mineral deficiencies you have.

Once you have your results, follow the instructions later in this chapter for introducing an elimination diet. Once you have completed this, move on to reintroducing certain foods. Finally, stick with a rotation diet so that the food intolerances do not return. You should start feeling a noticeable difference in your symptoms after eradicating the food intolerances.

Evaluate your Primary Health Puzzle Pieces (PHPPs) to determine whether anything is out of balance. Also refer to your Wheel of Digestive Health to see whether you would like to change any particular area of your life. Remember, food is filling, but not "fulfilling"; always consider that although food plays a huge role in IBD, managing your PHPPs is critical to your overall health and well-being. If an aspect of your Wheel of Digestive Health raises concerns, focus on improving this area of your life and see if your symptoms improve.

Score 40–58: High Priority

With a high-priority score, make no mistake—it is quite likely that you have a food intolerance. You may also be experiencing a bad flare-up, so contact your doctor if you feel your symptoms are becoming overwhelming. Trust your gut instinct.

Follow all the directions detailed for readers with a medium-priority score. However, if your symptoms are this severe, you may want to skip the food diary and just contact a health practitioner to order the Metametrix blood work. You may have multiple severe food intolerances and will undoubtedly need to follow an elimination diet in addition to completing the recommendations listed in the medium-priority section.

If you have a severe food intolerance, your body is producing antigens that place a significant amount of strain on your immune system. Food-intolerance reactions also cause your body to become riddled with inflammation because these harmful foods cause the production of cytokines. If your body is working overtime, you may need extra rest. You would also benefit from the use of supplements. Follow the recommended supplement protocol listed in Chapter 3 for at least six months to a year to improve your overall digestive physiology. This will give your gut a chance to heal while allowing your immune system to restore itself.

The Science Behind IBD and Food Intolerance

In the health world, the subject of food intolerance is a hot topic. Some practitioners embrace the concept, but some are still unsure of its validity. I acknowledge this split; however, more and more promising studies detail the benefits of identifying IgG food intolerance in patients with Crohn's and colitis. I will discuss several of these studies so you can understand how this research has contributed to the principles outlined in *The IBD Healing Plan and Recipe Book.*

A study titled "Clinical Relevance of IgG Antibodies Against Food Antigens in Crohn's Disease: A Double-Blind Cross-Over Intervention Study," published in a 2010 issue of *Digestion*, discovered that nutritional intervention based on circulating IgG antibodies against food antigens showed positive effects with respect to stool frequency. In other words, while refraining from consuming foods that caused a reaction, patients saw their bowel movements actually decrease. It further noted that abdominal pain was reduced and general well-being was improved. In a pilot study, seventy-nine Crohn's patients and twenty healthy controls were examined for IgG antibodies. Thereafter, the clinical relevance of these food IgG antibodies was assessed in a double-blind cross-over study with forty patients. Based on the presence of IgG antibodies, a nutritional intervention was planned. The pilot study resulted in a significant difference of IgG antibodies in serum between Crohn's patients and healthy controls. The vast majority of the patients produced IgG antibodies in response to the intake of processed cheese (84 percent) and yeast (83 percent). The daily stool frequency significantly decreased by 11 percent when following a specific diet that eliminated the processed cheese and yeast, compared to a sham diet.[4] This study indicates that examining the relationship between IgG food intolerance and IBD is valid.

A study published in *Human Nutrition: Applied Nutrition* found that an IgG food-intolerance immune-system reaction can occur in patients with Crohn's disease. In the study, twenty-nine of the thirty-three participants reported food intolerances. Those affected were instructed to follow an elimination diet. In the end, twenty-one of the twenty-nine food-intolerant patients remained in remission thanks to an adjusted diet alone for an average of 15.2 months.[5]

According to an article in *Food Matters* by Dr. Anton Emmanuel, consultant gastroenterologist and senior lecturer in neuro-gastroenterology at University College Hospital, London, several case studies on IBD patients were performed to determine whether a correlation between IBD and IgG food intolerance exists. Dr. Emmanuel reports, "Our group has shown that there are increased levels of food specific IgG antibodies in Crohn's disease compared to controls (participants who did not have the disease). These results suggest further experiments to investigate whether IgG antibodies can predict foods that provoke disease in double-blind, placebo-controlled food challenges and conversely, whether specific food avoidances based on antibody titres (tested levels) might be worthwhile."[6] Although there is not a terrible wealth of research out there yet, I wager that within the next couple of decades, this area of science will be studied much more explicitly and will prove its significance.

IBD Food Intolerance Case Study

Once I had discovered that my own case of Crohn's was aggravated by food intolerance, I began to question the role it played for others with IBD. I began a case study of my own and was shocked by the results. They suggested that inflammatory bowel disease can improve when IgG reactions are distinguished and reactive foods are eliminated from the patient's diet.

Do Food Intolerance and Stress Play a Role in IBD?

Purpose: The following case study details the effects of IgG food intolerance in patients with IBD or irritable bowel syndrome (IBS) and the direct role diet and lifestyle attributed to these illnesses. The study also aimed to determine whether a reduction in mental and physical stress reduced digestive distress. Each case presented with IBD, such as Crohn's, colitis, or celiac disease. It should be noted that some of the patients in the study had only IBS.

Study Group: The study included nineteen people from my private practice, ranging from a five-year-old boy to a sixty-seven-year-old woman.

Procedure: Each member of the group was tested for IgG food intolerance for up to ninety foods to determine the direct effects of cytokine production causing immune and inflammatory response in the gut. If food intolerance was present, the patient was asked to adhere to a strict elimination diet for at least thirty days, followed by a reintroduction period and a rotation diet, if necessary.

The subjects were then asked to limit stress and to participate in the Midwest Center for Stress and Anxiety Home program in conjunction with receiving nutrition and lifestyle counseling. Patients were encouraged to relax while eating (no reading or TV watching or eating lunch at their desks), to chew foods slowly, to eat organically, and to avoid foods that showed elevated antigen response, per the IgG testing.

Findings: The food-intolerance testing clearly indicated a relationship between cytokine production in the gut and the production of antigens due to inappropriate food consumption in IBD patients. Each participant tested positive for at least two food intolerances, with the highest number being forty-eight. The average number of food intolerances per person was ten, with five of those being severe. A reaction is classified as severe when the body produces more than two thousand antigens each time an offending food is consumed. These statistics suggest that food intolerance plays a role in IBD.

▌IgG Ninety Antigens Food-Intolerance Testing Results

SUBJECT	AGE	SEX	DIAGNOSIS	NUMBER OF FOOD INTOLERANCES	NUMBER OF SEVERE INTOLERANCES	SPECIFIC FOOD INTOLERANCES
A	5	Male	Crohn's	2	2	Gluten, casein, milk
B	8	Male	Autism, IBS	39	21	Too many to list
C	9	Male	Leaky gut, gut dysbiosis, IBS	48	33	Too many to list
D	11	Male	Crohn's	8	1	Casein, milk, eggs, gluten, soy, malt

(cont'd.)

▊ IgG Ninety Antigens Food-Intolerance Testing Results (cont'd.)

SUBJECT	AGE	SEX	DIAGNOSIS	NUMBER OF FOOD INTOLERANCES	NUMBER OF SEVERE INTOLERANCES	SPECIFIC FOOD INTOLERANCES
E	16	Female	Crohn's	6	5	Milk, eggs, vanilla, peanuts, soy
F	17	Male	Crohn's	3	3	Eggs, milk, casein, gluten
G	19	Male	Crohn's	6	2	Eggs, casein, milk, gluten, ginger
H	27	Female	Colitis	3	2	Casein, eggs, milk
I	27	Female	Colitis	12	3	Casein, eggs, milk, apples, cantaloupes, cranberries, lima beans, peanuts, mustard, cucumbers, almonds
J	31	Female	Crohn's	5	0	Ginger, milk, lactose, eggs, navy and pinto beans
K	38	Female	Crohn's	2	1	Gluten, fructose
L	39	Female	IBS	2	2	Gluten, casein, milk
M	45	Female	Colitis	5	3	Casein, milk, dairy, eggs, gluten, mustard
N	46	Female	IBS, MS	2	2	Casein, milk, gluten
O	53	Female	Crohn's	10	2	Casein, milk, gluten, navy and pinto beans, flounder, halibut, lobster, almonds, cashews
P	57	Female	Crohn's	13	5	Casein, eggs, milk, grapes, rye, wheat, navy and pinto beans, mushrooms, mustard, malt, sunflowers

(cont'd.)

▌IgG Ninety Antigens Food-Intolerance Testing Results (cont'd.)

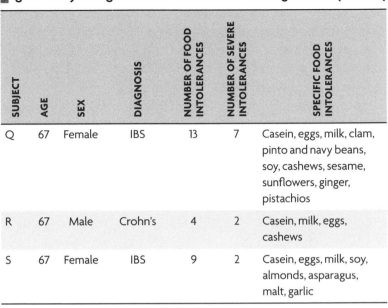

SUBJECT	AGE	SEX	DIAGNOSIS	NUMBER OF FOOD INTOLERANCES	NUMBER OF SEVERE INTOLERANCES	SPECIFIC FOOD INTOLERANCES
Q	67	Female	IBS	13	7	Casein, eggs, milk, clam, pinto and navy beans, soy, cashews, sesame, sunflowers, ginger, pistachios
R	67	Male	Crohn's	4	2	Casein, milk, eggs, cashews
S	67	Female	IBS	9	2	Casein, eggs, milk, soy, almonds, asparagus, malt, garlic

All participants were asked to keep a log of their daily stress levels. During the course of a thirty-day food-elimination program, seventeen of the nineteen participants recorded a reduction in stress levels once they abstained from eating foods they could not tolerate and began the Midwest center program. While completing this study, the participants also reported a significant increase in energy, vitality, and overall improved mood levels. From this, one could speculate that the phenomenon could have been due to increased levels of serotonin brought on by removing inflammatory agents that would diminish healthy bacteria flora in the gut. (Earlier in the book I touched on the connection between serotonin levels and digestion; see page 20.) Hormone levels were not tested, so the study is inconclusive on this point, but it serves as a possible hypothesis. All participants reported that chewing food more thoroughly and concentrating on digestion by omitting extraneous activity while eating, such as driving or watching TV, tremendously aided stress levels and eradicated bloating, pain, and digestive discomforts, such as flatulence and cramping.

Conclusion: A direct and concrete relationship exists between digestive distress and IgG food intolerances. Reducing stress and eliminating foods that cause stress to the body can have a profound effect on the body's ability to function optimally. All patients in the case study reported significant improvement in mood levels, energy, and decreased digestive distress.

Many more studies have been published on links between diet and IBD. You are probably aware of how important good nutrition is for treating any health ailment. Obviously, it is even more important to focus on diet if you have IBD. You should consider your digestive system a precious gift that allows you to enjoy certain foods and absorb nutrition. Your intestines are the guards for your immune system and should be well cared for to achieve optimal health.

Testing Methods for Food Intolerance

How can you determine whether you have a food intolerance? Two different methods are effective for diagnosing food intolerance: Requesting blood work or keeping a food diary. I recommend former if possible, because it is the most definite and accurate method for obtaining information. However, if your health-insurance provider won't cover blood work, you can keep the journal and then consult with a professional to help pinpoint any sensitivities. If you can do blood work, labs such as Metametrix, Genova Diagnostics, and ALCAT all provide testing for food intolerance. You can find more information about these labs in the Resources section.

The Food Diary

The food diary is a powerful tool for bringing awareness to your eating patterns. Feel free to use this form or recreate it in a more convenient way that works for you (such as in a notepad, in your day planner, or on your computer).

Note how you feel physically and emotionally before, during, and after each meal, snack, and beverage. At first it may feel odd to pay this much attention to your reactions, and it may be difficult to notice differences. That is okay—just write "fine" or "good." Take notice if your digestion changes and if you experience any food-intolerance symptoms, such as bloating, fatigue, abdominal cramping, or lack of energy. A score of 0 would indicate no digestive problems, and a score of 5 would indicate severe issues.

Once you have kept your food diary for three weeks, you should have a pretty good idea of whether food intolerance is contributing to your IBD. Consistent patterns will start to emerge. Look for commonalities with symptoms and a specific food group. For example, you drink milk on Monday and have a stomach attack, on Wednesday you have macaroni and cheese and have abnormal bowel movements, and on Thursday you have yogurt and break out in hives. These symptoms would point to a dairy intolerance. Pay special attention to some of the most common foods that IBD patients react to (as you can see in the study described on page 52), as these may be foods that cause reactions.

 If you are unable to distinguish a clear pattern, or if you are having trouble implementing this diary on your own, seek out a naturopath or nutritionist to help you. On many occasions, I have worked with clients with whom we were looking for a needle in a haystack, and we discovered some of the most innocent foods, such as mustard or sweet potatoes, were the culprits. Cases like this can be difficult to crack on your own, so visit nutrition professionals in your area who have experience with IBD and food intolerance.

The Digestion Diary

I find that many people are shocked once they look at what they consume on a daily basis. Some of us are creatures of habit and eat the same items over and over, while others are always trying new things. Please be mindful to bring this diary with you as you travel throughout your day. It is very important to be as accurate as possible when filling out the diary, so you can discover which food is causing a potential reaction.

▌My Digestion Diary

DATE/TIME	FOODS (PREPARATION, HOW MUCH)	WHERE (PLACE, ACTIVITY)	THOUGHTS (EMOTIONAL/ PHYSICAL/MOOD)
Breakfast			
Lunch			
PM/Snacks			
Dinner			
Evening Snack(s)			
Other			
Gum, Alcohol, Candy			

Blood Testing

One of the best testing methodologies for food intolerance available today is offered through Metametrix labs. If you suspect you have food intolerance, contact Metametrix for assistance locating a practitioner in your area who can order an IgG Food Antibody Blood Test. Once you have the results, you can begin to eliminate the foods that are likely contributing to your IBD. This method is preferred over the food diary because of its quick turnaround time and accuracy; results are usually available in about two weeks with Metametrix versus three weeks with the food diary.

The test measures the level of antigens present in your blood when it is exposed to certain food particles. The IgG profile tests for more than ninety different foods. The results show the number of IgG antibodies produced in response to each particular food. The numbers range from ten to two thousand (measured in nanograms per milliliter).

Here is a sample test so you can understand what results looks like. The box below categorizes the number of any antigens present when exposed to foods. The numbers are grouped into several categories, with +1 and +2 being mild, +3 and +4 being moderate, and +5 being severe sensitivity to that food. Each food has a number value listed next to it. If it is fewer than 10, the number indicates no food sensitivity. *If a food has forty or more antigens present, a sensitivity or intolerance is evident, and the food should therefore be omitted to avoid symptoms.* For example the subject in the test below has an intolerance to the following foods: barley, beef, casein, cashews, chicken, clam, crab, eggs, garlic, lamb, lentils, lobster, malt, milk, mustard, oranges, oyster, peanuts, peas, pistachios, pork, rye, salmon, sesame, shrimp, soy, turkey, and wheat.

The patient should refrain from eating these foods for at least thirty days and then carefully reintroduce the foods later. This is because for some people, clearing the problematic food from the diet for period of time allows the gut to heal, and as a result, a once-reactive food ceases to cause problems. This does not always happen, but it can. If you reintroduce a food and find that you are no longer intolerant of it, you can follow a rotation diet (see page 69) to ensure the food intolerance does not return.

Sample IgG Food Antibody Test

NUMBER OF ANTIGENS	CLASS OF REACTION
0–40*	Negative
80–150	Mild (+1/+2)
500–900	Moderate (+3/+4)
1,000–2,000	Severe (+5)

* While some antigens might be present, if the number is under 40 the reaction isn't severe enough to warrant eliminating a food from your diet.

▌Sample IgG Food Antibody Test (cont'd.)

FOOD GROUP/FOOD	ANTIGENS	REACTION CLASS
Dairy/Meat/Poultry		
Beef	60	Mild +1
Casein	>2,000	Severe +5
Chicken	126	Mild +2
Egg, white	>2,000	Severe +5
Egg, yolk	728	Mod +4
Lamb	209	Mod +3
Milk	>2,000	Severe +5
Pork	74	Mild +1
Turkey	232	Mod +3
Grains		
Barley	238	Mod +3
Corn	<10	
Oat	<10	
Rice	<10	
Rye	434	Mod +3
Wheat	1,458	Severe +5
Fish/Shellfish		
Clam	80	Mild +1
Codfish	22	
Crab	285	Mod +3
Flounder	30	
Halibut	36	
Lobster	505	Mod +4
Mackerel	<10	
Oyster	642	Mod +4
Salmon	44	Mild +1
Shrimp	749	Mod +4
Tuna	30	

(cont'd.)

▌Sample IgG Food Antibody Test (cont'd.)

FOOD GROUP/FOOD	ANTIGENS	REACTION CLASS
Trout	30	
Legumes		
Green pea	146	Mild +2
Lentil	251	Mod +3
Lima bean	<10	
Navy bean	38	
Peanut	>2000	Severe +5
Pinto bean	12	
Soybean	953	Severe +5
String bean	32	
Nuts/Seeds		
Almond	<10	
Cashew	473	Mod +3
Coconut	14	
Pecan	<10	
Pistachio	402	Mod +3
Sesame	46	Mild +1
Sunflower	17	
Walnut	16	
Vegetables		
Asparagus	<10	
Avocado	<10	
Broccoli	<10	
Cabbage	18	
Carrot	<10	
Cauliflower	30	
Celery	<10	
Cucumber	<10	
Garlic	626	Mod +4

(cont'd.)

▍Sample IgG Food Antibody Test (cont'd.)

FOOD GROUP/FOOD	ANTIGENS	REACTION CLASS
Green pepper	20	
Lettuce	<10	
Mushroom	16	
Mustard	926	Severe +5
Olive	<10	
Onion	16	
Potato	<10	
Spinach	<10	
Sweet potato	10	
Tomato	<10	
Zucchini	12	
Fruits		
Apple	<10	
Apricot	<10	
Banana	17	
Blueberry	<10	
Cantaloupe	9	
Cranberry	20	
Grape	<10	
Grapefruit	35	
Honeydew	<10	
Lemon	<10	
Orange	109	Mild +2
Peach	<10	
Pear	30	
Pineapple	24	
Strawberry	10	
Watermelon	13	

(cont'd.)

▌Sample IgG Food Antibody Test (cont'd.)

FOOD GROUP/FOOD	ANTIGENS	REACTION CLASS
Miscellaneous		
Aspergillus	<10	
Black pepper	<10	
Chocolate	17	
Cinnamon	<10	
Coffee	23	
Ginger	12	
Malt	411	Mod +3
Tea	<10	
Vanilla	<10	
Yeast, baker's	11	
Yeast, brewer's	8	

The Food-Elimination Diet

To complete an elimination diet, you remove all offending foods that were reported in the IgG food antibody profile (or your food journal) for at least ninety days. This applies to all foods that cause a reaction, regardless of the severity. During this time, you will also perform an overhaul of your diet. Ideally you should encourage your whole family to participate, which increases your potential to remain compliant. As you can imagine, this process requires constant monitoring of your diet. Rest assured, your efforts will be greatly rewarded.

In addition to the suspect foods, you must also eliminate:

- junk foods—Including fast foods, candy, sodas, cookies, cakes, and refined sugars
- processed foods—Including pressed meats and cheeses
- food additives—This requires checking labels very carefully. Avoid products that have long ingredient lists, as they are likely to include preservatives, coloring, and/or artificial flavors, all of which should be avoided. Beware of any ingredients

containing the words "agent," "enhancer," "sodium benzoate," "nitrate," "regulator," "bleach," and "gums," or any ingredients ending in "-ant." Even foods containing natural flavors may not be safe, as they may contain monosodium glutamate, or MSG, a powerful excitotoxin (a class of substances that damages neurons) capable of passing through the blood–brain barrier.

- trans fats—Beware of foods that contain hydrogenated fats or oils. These are used in packaged foods to preserve the shelf life. At the time of this writing, trans fats are banned in Europe and in all New York City and Long Island restaurants. I suspect this positive trend will increase as time goes on.

Add more organic foods to your diet, eliminating pesticides, growth hormones, genetically modified organisms, fungicides, and irradiation.

Withdrawal Symptoms

You may experience some withdrawal as a result of eliminating some foods, but these symptoms should subside within two weeks.

Possible symptoms include:

- cheating on the elimination diet
- depression
- difficulty sleeping
- irritability
- lethargy

When the diet is followed correctly, you will see a significant improvement in general health and IBD symptoms in four to twelve weeks. If you do not, it means one of the following:

- You ate off-limit foods without your knowledge.
- The food(s) you are sensitive to has not been identified yet.
- You may not have designed the elimination diet properly. Try doing it again and remove more foods.
- You knowingly cheated on the diet.
- The foods you eat are not actually contributing to your IBD.

If this happens, you must start over again, so be careful! Even the smallest amount of an offending food can set you back.

 To properly set up the diet, map out your plan *prior* to embarking upon this lifestyle change. To feel more comfortable with the changes, try at least a few new recipes that include acceptable, new foods. Stock your kitchen properly with ingredients that are tolerable. For example, ensure you have gluten-free/dairy-free bread in the house so you are not scrambling around at dinnertime looking for it. Keeping organized will lead to success and far less stress. Many patients understandably try to master their plans for the elimination diet in a few hours, but this is not realistic. Don't set yourself up for failure. Give yourself a week to stock your pantry and to create a menu plan with appropriate foods for the coming week. Once these tasks are completed, *only then* should you move forward with your elimination diet. You will be glad that you planned ahead.

The Reintroduction Diet

After twelve weeks on the elimination diet, you can start to slowly reintroduce foods that were off limits. This can take one to six weeks depending on how many foods you need to reintroduce (see "Smart Tip" below). Begin adding eliminated foods one at a time, in no particular order. However, you should avoid indulging in the food you are craving the most until all others have been tried. Typically, the most desired food is the kind that you have become addicted to, and reintroducing it will likely cause a noticeable reaction. Reintroduction takes at least three days per food, and sometimes longer depending on whether you experience a reaction.

 The reintroduction of foods can take anywhere from a week to several weeks, depending on how many food sensitivities you have. For example, if you have three food sensitivities and it takes at least three days to reintroduce each offending food, your elimination diet would take at least nine days.

Reintroduction-Diet Guidelines

Reintroduce each food for one day only, with increasing amounts consumed at each meal throughout that day. Then remove the food from your diet again. Observe your reactions for seventy-two hours. *If you do not experience a reaction,* move on to the next food. *If you do experience a reaction,* wait until it has ceased and you have had no symptoms for twenty-four hours before moving on to the next food.

Record the quantity of the food eaten and the time of day in your "Food Reintroduction Chart" (see page 68).

Record all the symptoms that you observe, the time they occurred, and their duration.

At the beginning of each day, make a note in the diary regarding the quality of your sleep the night before and your general behavior the previous day (lethargy, moodiness, stuffy nose, and so forth).

If you suffer from a flare-up, cold, or infection during this process, suspend the food reintroduction until after recovery, and continue the elimination diet.

Question: What types of symptoms should you look for when you reintroduce a food?

Answer: One of the top questions my clients ask me is, "How can I tell if I have had a reaction to a food?" There are a number of symptoms you can look for that indicate a reaction, and I will break them down for you below. However, keep in mind that sometimes it can be tricky to identify a reaction for a couple of reasons.

1. It is easy to take your "tell-tale" symptoms for granted, especially when you have IBD. Instead of viewing ongoing symptoms as a warning sign, many patients tell me, "I am used to my symptoms. I have simply found a way to cope with them." Even if you think your body is accustomed to symptoms, it is really trying to *tell you something*—that your balance has been altered to some degree.

2. Since it can take up to seventy-two hours for a reaction to a food to occur, I recommend you write down how you feel after each meal. Most people would not normally think that a reaction on Wednesday could be attributed to a food con-

sumed on Monday, but this can and does happen, which is why keeping a food diary is very important.

How Can You Tell If You Have a Reaction to a Food?

As you become more conscious of the foods you consume on a daily basis by journaling, you will begin to observe different indicators of health through signs of physical and emotional balance. This discovery can be a gradual process for most, which is why it is a great idea to write everything down in your food diary. You will likely forget how you felt after breakfast three days ago, and this lack of recollection can alter the results of your reintroduction and food challenge.

Balanced Physical and Emotional Symptoms

Clues for balance can be physical and emotional in nature. Physical balance includes feeling appropriate hunger, displaying adequate stamina, experiencing natural deep breathing, and having high energy, restful sleep, sufficient and comfortable focus, alertness, agility, good attention span, and good color. If your body is in a healthy state, you should enjoy these excellent physical traits. If you have good emotional balance, you should feel confident, excited, energized, humorous, happy, interested, focused, calm, relaxed, easygoing, and patient.

Physical and Emotional Signs to Look For

If a reaction is triggered in you as an IBD patient, how will you feel *physically?* Those who suffer from food intolerance report various physical symptoms, including headaches, stomach pain, insomnia, muscle cramps, coughing, fatigue, restlessness, shakiness, muscle weakness, poor concentration, and/or pallor (paleness). *Emotional symptoms may be a little harder to notice.* Clues for emotional imbalance include feeling anxious, bored, scared, mad, sad, depressed, scattered, restless, irritable, agitated, or hyper.

If you experience any indications of imbalance after you have reintroduced a food, you are still sensitive to it and should avoid this food. If you have a reaction immediately after eating a reintroduced food, do not continue eating it. You have gotten your answer and can now take the item back out of your diet. The physical and emotional symptoms listed above should be watched for after you eat to determine whether the food being reintroduced is still causing a problem. Keep accurate notes, as this process is going to help you formulate a long-term diet.

Reintroduction Results

You should have clearly observed that certain symptoms subsided while you were on the elimination diet and returned when a certain food or foods were reintroduced. These suspects should be considered food sensitivities, and you should completely abandon them until you have been symptom-free for at least one year.

Sometimes food sensitivities can eradicate themselves if the offending food is not consumed for a period of time. This is not always the case, but it can be a pleasant surprise. If a genetic predisposition makes you unable to break down the food, unfortunately, you have no other solution but to avoid the food permanently.

If you are reintroducing a food and are not sure whether you have had a reaction, try reintroducing the food again a few weeks later. This can happen more with children, who have more of a tendency to have a behavioral "meltdown" when reintroduced to offending foods. However, if a child has a perceived reaction to a food on the same day that they have a fight with their best friend, it is not likely you could distinguish the root cause of the reaction. In this situation, wait and try the food again in a few weeks.

Sample Food Reintroduction Chart

DATE	FOOD	REACTION
Jan 1	Wheat	Experienced mild reaction. Headache. Reaction began on Jan 2 and lasted one day. Symptom free on Jan 3. Move to next food Jan 4.
Jan 4	Eggs	No reaction observed.
Jan 8	Milk	No reaction observed.

The Rotation Diet

Remember, the reintroduction diet is designed to determine if you are still reacting to foods that either have been identified via blood work as problematic or that you suspect are causing your IBD to flare-up. Once you have completed the reintroduction diet, the rotation diet is your next step. For example, if you initially found yourself being intolerant to dairy but did not see any symptoms when you reintroduced it, you could then put dairy into a rotation diet. A rotation diet allows you to rotate the once forbidden food back into your elimination diet, allowing you to eat the food once every four days or so. The table below provides a sample menu for a dairy, gluten, and egg rotation diet. Notice how each one of these foods in only eaten once every four days. This is what you are looking to do for yourself.

Why should you eat this way? When the same food is eaten over and over again, it can cause an immune reaction that can lead to the creation of a food sensitivity. After all of your hard work on the elimination diet and reintroduction, we wouldn't want the food sensitivity to reoccur. The purpose of a rotation diet is to allow you to resume eating these foods, but only occasionally. Most people tend to repeatedly eat the things they like, which is not good. In the nutrition field, professionals constantly stress variety to ensure you are getting well-rounded nutrition. For example, if you were to eat apples and green beans daily and avoid other foods, you would eventually be deficient in many things. I have also found in clinical practice that people who eat the same foods again and again are more likely to have an IgG reaction show up with the food they eat most often in addition to having vitamin and mineral deficiencies.

Rotation Diet Rules

A rotation diet follows a four-day cycle. You'll vary foods within the same food family for four days and then start over again. Use plenty of variety to ensure you are getting enough vegetables, fruits, and protein-rich foods daily for optimal nutrition.

Remember to do the following:

- Read all food labels and become familiar with the many names a food may be called.

- When shopping and cooking, keep in mind that many commercially prepared foods and supplements have hidden additives used as fillers, such as wheat, yeast, or egg byproducts.

- Keep a food symptoms journal, including time, amount, and any changes in attitude, alertness, aches, pains, skin, pulse, hearing, vision, and fatigue.

- Do not feel that you have to prepare more than one diet in your household. The rotation plan can benefit the whole family by decreasing the likelihood of developing food reactions.

- Include at least three different food groups at each meal.

- Avoid consuming canned, packaged, or fast foods. They contain many hidden and possibly allergenic (IgE food allergy) constituents and often lack wholesome ingredients.

- Unrefined, cold pressed oils are preferred (olive, sesame, coconut). Use organic brands when possible.

- Try to relax and chew, so the food is broken down for easier digestion.

Example of Dairy-, Wheat-, and Egg-Free 4-Day Rotation Diet

	Breakfast	Lunch	Dinner
DAY 1	• Buckwheat cereal with soymilk • Clementine slices • Banana	• Grilled chicken breast with pineapple slices • Baked sweet potato • Streamed Brussels sprouts	• Tofu and vegetable (spinach, carrots, celery) stir-fry over millet • Water
DAY 2	• Brown rice with raisins • Chopped walnuts • Rice milk • Blueberries	• Roasted turkey • Spaghetti squash • Cucumber dill salad • Peppermint tea	• Steak and vegetables (bamboo shoots, mushrooms, zucchini) over wild rice • Mango slices • Coconut water

(cont'd.)

Example of Dairy-, Wheat-, and Egg-Free 4-Day Rotation Diet (cont'd.)

	Breakfast	Lunch	Dinner
DAY 3	• Gluten-free corn bread toast, cashew butter, butter • Kiwis • Chamomile tea	• Salmon • Steamed broccoli • Pear slices and almonds	• Grilled white fish tacos • Shredded romaine • Avocado • Whole-grain corn shell • Rice • Cheese (optional) • Carrot juice
DAY 4	• Wheat toast with apricot preserves • Fruit salad of plums and cherries • pau d'arco tea	• Sesame tuna with soy sauce • Grilled asparagus • Quinoa cranberry pilaf	• Tomato sauce with wheat pasta • Artichoke • Peaches • Water

Grocery Shopping Cards

Whether you are on an elimination diet, reintroduction diet, or rotation diet, shopping can get a little tricky in some cases. Therefore, I have included an invaluable resource to instantly make your trips to the grocery store easier. Here are some substitutions for the eight most common allergens. When you are shopping and are unsure of what products you can use as substitutions, refer to these lists for help.

Print these cards on heavy paper, cut them out, and place them in your wallet or purse. Ideally, you should print the substitutions on one side of the card and the foods to watch out for on the other.

SUBSTITUTIONS FOR CORN

VEGETABLES

- acorn squash
- beans
- buttercup squash
- butternut squash
- banana
- carrots
- eggplants
- peas
- peppers
- pumpkins
- red peppers
- sweet potatoes
- tomatoes
- yams
- yellow squash
- winter squash

GRAINS

- amaranth
- barley
- buckwheat
- kamut
- millet
- quinoa
- rice
- teff

THICKENERS

- arrowroot
- kuzu
- potato starch
- tapioca starch

SNACKS OR SIDES

- Clif Bars
- Enjoy Life Bars
- flour tortillas
- Lara Bars
- rice crackers and cakes

HOW TO AVOID CORN IN PRODUCTS

CORN MAY BE LISTED ON LABELS AS:

- baking powder
- glucose syrup
- high-fructose corn syrup
- hominy
- maize
- masa harina
- starch—cereal, corn, food, modified
- vegetable—gum, protein, paste, starch

FOODS LIKELY TO CONTAIN CORN

- baked goods
- beverages and alcohol
- candies
- canned fruits
- cereals
- cookies
- deli meats
- grits
- hominy
- infant formulas
- jams and jellies
- popcorn
- snack foods
- syrups
- other convenience foods

‹‹ available for download at www.hunterhouse.com ››

SUBSTITUTES FOR PEANUTS

NUTS/SEEDS

- almonds
- Brazil nuts
- cashews
- pecans

- pine nuts
- pistachios
- pumpkin seeds
- soy nuts

- sunflower seeds
- walnuts

NUT BUTTERS

- almond
- cashew
- sesame

HOW TO AVOID PEANUTS IN PRODUCTS

PLEASE AVOID...

- arachis oil
- beer nuts
- goober nuts
- groundnuts
- mandelonas
- mixed nuts
- monkey nuts

- nu-nuts
- nutmeat
- nut pieces
- peanutamide
- peanuts
- peanut butter

- peanut oil (cold pressed, expelled, or extruded)
- peanut sprouts
- peanut flour
- sodium peanutate

PEANUTS CAN BE FOUND IN...

- African dishes
- Asian/Indian dishes
- biscuits
- breakfast cereals
- chocolates
- dried fruit mixes
- gravy

- health-food bars
- ice creams
- lollipops and hard candy
- marzipan
- Mexican dishes
- nougat

- praline
- pesto salad/salad dressing
- sauces
- snack foods
- soup

‹‹ available for download at www.hunterhouse.com ››

SUBSTITUTIONS FOR DAIRY

MILK

• homemade potato milk	(does not contain THC)	vanilla, chocolate)
• Hood Almond Milk	• Nature's Promise	• Pacific Natural Foods Almond Milk
• Native Forest Organic Coconut Milk	Rice Milk (plain, vanilla, chocolate)	(vanilla, chocolate)
• Native Forest Organic Hemp Milk	• Nature's Promise Soy Milk (plain,	• Silk Soy Milk (plain, vanilla, chocolate)

BUTTER

• coconut butter (works well for baking)	• Earth Balance Spread	• Willow Run Soybean Margarine Stick

CHEESE

• cheese: edam, cheddar, mozzarella, and blue	• Daiya Mozzarella Cheese	• Redwood Gouda Style Cheese
• Daiya Cheddar Cheese	• Provamel Dairy-Free Spread (Cheddar and Garlic)	• Tofutti Vegan Crème Cheese
		• Vegan Parma

YOGURT/ICE CREAM

• frozen bananas dipped in organic dark chocolate	• So Delicious Coconut Ice Cream	• Tofutti Ice Cream
• So Delicious Coconut-Based Yogurt (assorted flavors, including vanilla, raspberry, blueberry)	• So Delicious Soy-Based Yogurt (assorted flavors, including blueberry, vanilla, mango)	• Tofutti Soy Ice Cream Sandwiches
	• Sorbet	• Water Ices from Ralph's Italian Ice

‹‹ available for download at www.hunterhouse.com ››

HOW TO AVOID DAIRY IN PRODUCTS

PLEASE AVOID...

- butter and many margarines
- canned foods (soups, spaghetti, ravioli)
- cream soups and chowders
- cream, cheese, or butter sauces (often on vegetables or meats)

- macaroni and cheese
- many "nondairy" products (coffee creamer, whipped toppings)
- many baked goods (bread, crackers, desserts)
- many baking mixes (pancake mix)

- many salad dressings (ranch, blue cheese, creamy, Caesar)
- mashed potatoes (often prepared with butter and/or milk)
- shakes and hot chocolate mixes and drinks

HOW TO READ DAIRY ON LABELS

- butter or artificial-butter flavor
- buttermilk or buttermilk solids
- casein, caseinate, sodium caseinate (check lab results for +casein)

- cheese, cream cheese, cottage cheese
- cream, sour cream, half and half, whipped cream
- lactose, lactalbumin

- milk, milk solids, nonfat milk solids
- whey
- yogurt, kefir

DAIRY-FREE SOURCES OF CALCIUM

- almonds
- beans (kidney, pinto, navy, soy)
- broccoli
- calcium-fortified rice milk
- calcium-fortified orange juice

- canned salmon with bones
- figs
- green, leafy vegetables (kale, spinach, romaine lettuce)
- molasses
- rhubarb

- sardines
- soy products, such as tofu, tempeh, and calcium-fortified soymilk

« available for download at www.hunterhouse.com »

SUBSTITUTIONS FOR EGGS

- ENER-G® egg replacement powder
- 1 tbsp baking powder + 1 tsp gelatin + 2 tbsp flour = 1 egg (for puddings and custards)
- 2 tbsp water + ½ tsp oil + ½ tsp baking powder + 2 tbsp water = 1 egg
- 1 tbsp vegetable oil + ½ tsp baking powder = 1 egg

- 1 tbsp flaxseed powder + 3 tbsp warm water = 1 egg
- 1 tbsp gelatin or 1 tbsp fruit pectin (Sure Gel®) + 3 tbsp warm water = 1 egg
- Nonfat yogurt, mashed banana, applesauce, pumpkin, or other puréed fruit or vegetables are good replacements

for eggs in muffins or cakes. A half cup of puréed fruit or veggie equals one egg.
- To replace eggs in casseroles, burgers, or loaves, try mashed vegetables, tahini (sesame seed paste), nut butters, or rolled oats.

HOW TO AVOID EGG PRODUCTS

- albumin
- egg protein
- egg white
- egg yolk

- globulin
- livetin
- ovalbumin
- ovomucin

- ovomucoid
- ovovitellin
- powdered egg
- vitellin

FOODS LIKELY TO CONTAIN EGG...

- baked goods
- batter mixes
- Bavarian cream
- boiled dressing
- bouillon
- breaded foods
- breads
- cake flours
- creamy fillings
- custards
- egg-drop soup

- flan
- french toast
- fritters
- frosting
- hollandaise sauce
- ice cream
- macaroons
- malted drinks
- marshmallows
- mayonnaise
- meat loaf

- meringues
- noodles
- pancakes
- puddings
- quiche
- salad dressings
- sauces
- sausages
- soufflé
- tartar sauce
- waffles

《 available for download at www.hunterhouse.com 》

SUBSTITUTIONS FOR WHEAT/GLUTEN

BREADS

- Alexia's Bread Crumbs
- Alexia's Stuffing Mix
- Dr. Katz Gluten-Free Breads
- Ener-G Brown Rice Bread

- Enjoy Life Bread, Bagels
- Joan's Gluten-Free Great Bakes—Bagels, English Muffins, Pizza Crust
- Kinnikinnick Light Italian Bread, Bagels, Pizza Crust

- Pamela's Gluten-Free Corn Bread Mix
- Van's Gluten-Free Waffles

PASTA

- Chinese rice noodles (great for stir-fries)
- corn lasagna

- DeBoles Brown Rice Pasta
- Ancient Harvest Quinoa Pasta

- Mrs. Leeper's Gluten-Free Dinner Kits (Tuna Casserole, Mexican Beef Fiesta)

PASTRIES/DOUGHNUTS/COOKIES

- Annie's Vanilla Chocolate Bunny Cookies
- Betty Crocker G-F Brownie Mix
- Betty Crocker G-F Cake Mixes
- Cherrybrook Farms Vanilla/Chocolate Cake mix

- Dr. Katz Rainbow Vanilla Cookies
- Ener-G Cookies (Chocolate Crème)
- Glutino Pretzels
- Glutino Saltine Crackers
- Jo-Sef Vanilla Crème Cookies

- Kinnikinnick Doughnuts (vanilla, cinnamon sugar, chocolate)
- Pamela's Chocolate Chip Pancake Mix
- Pamela's Brownie Mix

Cut out card and affix to the card on the next page entitled "How to Avoid Wheat/Gluten Products" for a complete grocery list.

‹‹ available for download at www.hunterhouse.com ››

HOW TO AVOID WHEAT/GLUTEN PRODUCTS

PLEASE AVOID...

- baked goods, baking mixes (cakes, cookies, biscuits)
- beer and whiskey
- breaded and battered foods
- Carnation Instant Breakfast, malted and Postum drinks
- cereals
- crackers, pretzels, and other snack foods
- dumplings, croquettes, or patties
- gravies and sauces thickened with flour
- ice cream cones
- luncheon meats (bologna, ham) and meat loaf
- pancakes, waffles, doughnuts, muffins, crepes, and some corn breads
- pasta and noodles
- some soups and bouillon cubes
- soy sauce
- wheat-flour tortillas

HOW TO READ GLUTEN/WHEAT ON LABELS

Cereal binder	Usually wheat
Cereal filler	Usually wheat
Cereal protein	Usually wheat
Cereal starch	Usually wheat
Edible starch	Usually wheat or corn
Modified starch	Usually wheat or corn
Starch	Usually wheat or corn

The protein gluten is found in wheat, rye, barley, bulgur, spelt, triticale, malt, semolina, and durum flour, and oats (oats are contaminated with gluten, but by themselves don't contain it). If you are on a gluten-free diet, you must avoid these grains.

‹‹ available for download at www.hunterhouse.com ››

SUBSTITUTIONS FOR SOY

DAIRY

- Galaxy Food Vegan Rice Cheese—cheddar, mozzarella, pepper jack
- organic almond milk

- organic coconut milk
- organic cow's milk (preferably raw)
- organic goat's milk (preferably raw)

- organic rice milk
- So Delicious Coconut Yogurts

LEGUMES AND BEANS

- adzuki bean
- black bean
- black-eyed pea
- butter bean
- carob
- chickpea
- fava bean
- garbanzo bean

- green bean
- green pea
- kidney bean
- lentil
- lima bean
- navy bean
- northern bean
- peanut

- pinto bean
- snap bean, string bean
- snow pea
- split pea
- white bean

FLOUR

- amaranth
- barley
- buckwheat
- corn

- kamut
- lentil
- potato
- quinoa

- rice
- spelt
- tapioca
- teff

≪ available for download at www.hunterhouse.com ≫

HOW TO AVOID SOY IN PRODUCTS

PLEASE AVOID...

- canned foods (soups, spaghetti, ravioli)*
- cream soups and chowders
- many baked goods (bread, crackers, desserts)*
- many baking mixes (pancake mix)*
- many "nondairy" products (coffee creamer, whipped topping)
- many salad dressings (for example, Wishbone brand uses soybean oil instead of olive oil)
- miso soup
- So Delicious Soy Yogurt
- some dietary supplements (vitamin E, specifically)
- soy butter margarines
- soy cheese
- soy macaroni and cheese
- soy sauce
- tofu

*Beware of "low-quality," processed, or nonorganic foods that contain soy when they should not, such as Campbell's soup or Hostess brownies.

READING SOY ON LABELS...

- edamame
- hydrogenated soybean oil
- miso
- natto
- okara
- shoyu
- soya or soy lecithin
- tamari
- tempeh
- tofu (soybean curds)
- vegetable protein
- yuba

《 available for download at www.hunterhouse.com 》

Chapter 3

. . . .

Now That I Know I Have IBD, Which Foods Can Affect Me?

Food can be your friend or your enemy when you have inflammatory bowel disease (IBD), especially if you are unsure of what is affecting you. This chapter highlights foods that can have a negative effect on IBD. It is vital for you to become more conscious of these "problem foods" so you can abstain from them. This chapter teaches you the basics and is crucial to understanding how nutrition affects you. It even gives you the skinny on such hot nutrition topics as sugar and caffeine and their effects on the body especially as they relate to Crohn's, colitis, and celiac.

Steve's Story

The first time I spoke with Steve's mom, Suzy, she was pretty frustrated. Her thirteen-year-old son had been suffering from colitis for just over six months before she came into my practice. Suzy had taken her son to two pediatric gastroenterologists who had "dismissed" diet as a factor in his case. Mom did not agree, knowing Steve's diet was a little less than perfect. So after speaking with two of my former IBD clients, she decided to call me.

In our initial conversation, the concerned mother revealed that she and her husband, Bill, had not been satisfied with the answers they had been given about Steve's illness. According to Steve's doctors only medication or surgery would help. Steve had tried a few different medications for colitis, including Pentasa and Entocort, but they had been of little or no help. Suzy was quite worried, because Steve frequently ran fevers and was constantly run down and tired, causing him to start missing school.

Even on medications, Steve still averaged between six and eight bowel movements per day, and Suzy reported the odor to be offensive at times. I always joke with my IBD patients about using your "stool as a tool," because bodily waste can reveal so much about your health. So I asked Steve detailed questions about his "number 2" experiences. For instance, did his stool float or sink in the toilet? (Floating stool can indicate that undigested fat is present, which can be a sign of a metabolic issue.) Steve's stools did not sink, so he likely had an issue breaking down fats. The odor of the stool told me Steve either had toxins or bad bacteria overgrowth, or perhaps both.

I ran bloodwork, and, sure enough, both were problems. More important, though, was Steve's diet: It consisted of very typical, standard American fare, such as hot dogs, pizza, tacos, and an extraordinary amount of white foods, including breads, cookies, and pastas. What was even more alarming was that Steve had not consumed fruits and vegetables *at all* since he was a baby/toddler. His diet consisted solely of proteins and refined carbohydrates. It was the standard American diet at its "finest." I knew this was causing some major problems, because Steve's diet actually significantly promoted inflammation. In addition, his diet contained almost no macronutrients. He was pretty malnourished and lacked the naturally occurring probiotics, enzymes, fiber, phytochemicals, and phytonutrients that only plant-based foods can provide.

The highest priority was to adjust my young client's diet by adding whole foods, such as fruits and vegetables. The second items on Steve's wellness agenda included adding probiotics to fight off bad bacteria, conducting a juice cleanse to detoxify, and introducing a customized vitamin and amino acid (based off the results of a urinalysis). We worked slowly over five months to rebuild Steve's diet, adding broccoli, zucchini, apples, peppers, carrots, onions, bananas, and blueberries. He had many aversions to foods (typical among quite a few of my IBD clients), so I knew we had to slowly incorporate these items so that he would not regress back to his previous anti-fruit-and-vegetable diet. Thankfully, not only did he keep his new foods, he kept expanding from there. At the appointment that signified our five-month anniversary of nutrition counseling, he had not had a fever in three weeks, the putrid stools had ceased, his energy levels had climbed, and his complexion had transformed from pasty white to healthy and pink.

What was even more amazing to witness was the change in his bloodwork. His latest CBC (complete blood count), which measures the amounts of red and white blood cells in the body to indicate immune response, was normal for the first time. Suzy, Bill, and Steve were beyond thrilled. Thirteen is a tough age to make changes to the diet, but Steve did it so well that he put his disease in remission, where it has stayed.

Food Politics

After reading the previous chapter, you may have uncovered hidden food intolerances that contribute to your IBD. This close inspection of your former daily diet, especially if you have anything in common with Steve, may inspire you to start looking at food consumption in our society in a different light.

When I work with clients who suffer from IBD, it is usually because I am the person people reach out to after "everything else has failed," which mirrors my own history. Usually, people are intrigued by the term "holistic nutrition" but are not sure what it means. To better explain holistic nutrition's approach as opposed to conventional nutrition's, one of the first things I show clients is the USDA MyPlate (see Figure 2 below) and the Primary Health Puzzle Pieces (PHPPs) from Chapter 1 (see page 17). If you are looking for a general nutrition guide, the USDA Plate provides this in a small way by displaying the basic food groups: protein, fruits, vegetables, dairy, grains. However, one major factor that must be considered is the fact that each individual is

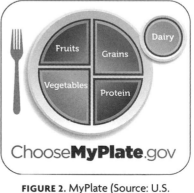

FIGURE 2. MyPlate (Source: U.S. Department of Agriculture)

different: No two people have the same lifestyle, ancestry, blood type, health conditions, DNA, and so forth. Given these unique traits, especially if you have IBD, how can the USDA Plate help you figure out if what you're eating today is right for you? Your PHPP exercises can assist you in examining these factors along with your lifestyle so that you can determine which foods are right for you.

What is strange is the large role given to the dairy group. Although calcium is found in many other foods, why is dairy food listed as the primary source when it is less healthy in many ways than vegetables? Food politics are likely at play here...

A study published in the *Journal of the American Dietetic Association* reported that 75 percent of adults worldwide lose their ability to digest lactose (the sugar found in dairy products) after infancy. The study went on to establish that lactose intolerance became more prevalent as the subjects entered adulthood.[1] What's even stranger is that we are one of the only cultures that continue to drink milk as we mature, and it comes from another animal. If you were not accustomed to this, would you feel this sounds bizarre?

Dairy is a particular concern for those with IBD, specifically Crohn's disease. In a study published by the *American Journal of Epidemiology*, a relationship was found between milk tainted with *Mycobacterium avium paratuberculosis* (MAP), a bacteria responsible for Johne's disease, a condition with symptoms similar to those of Crohn's that causes chronic inflammation and fatal intestinal disease in several domestic animals, especially dairy cows.[2] Internationally recognized Crohn's disease expert Dr. Jon Hermon-Taylor and several other researchers believe MAP, which is transferable through bovine milk and contaminated water, is responsible for the Crohn's disease epidemic.

I have always found the whole thing a bit odd. If evidence shows that patients with IBD cannot eat dairy, then why does the standard American diet encourage us to eat such a large quantity of these foods?

If you have embarked upon an elimination diet for your IBD, undoubtedly you have found that many of your favorite foods contain potential allergens. In turn, you may be wondering why the eight most common allergens are so prevalent in our diet today. Think about it: Wheat, soy, eggs, dairy, and nuts are in practically *everything*. The USDA-recommended foods are healthy for some people because they contain essential vitamins and nutrients, but the problem is that we have been taught that we should all eat the same things. Nothing could be further from the truth, especially if you suffer from IBD. No two human beings are exactly alike, and therefore no two diets should be the same.

At one time, good nutrition appeared straightforward and simple. Your great-grandmother knew best: "Sugar is bad, an apple a day is good, and don't forget your veggies" are some concrete words of wisdom she may have shared. These words were true then and are still true today. As a society, why does it seem as if we are so confused about how to eat? Books on diet and wellness are among the most popular sold today, because our culture is starving for the right information.

Part of the confusion stems from the fact that concepts about good nutrition tend to be influenced by corporations' agendas to sell foods. Sadly, food companies are not all concerned about promoting health. They are businesses. Their interest is selling you products, not necessarily enhancing your nutrition. Problems have existed in our system dating back all the way to 1894, when the USDA released its first attempt at dietary guidelines. And even though there is a wealth of information available today and the USDA has given us MyPlate (the 2011 revised guidelines meant to replace the food pyramid), the USDA continues to ignore the research proving that Americans eat excessive amounts of fats and sugar.[3]

What's even more interesting is that according to Marion Nestle, head of Public Nutrition at New York University, the food industry is not playing fair. In 1992 the first USDA food pyramid created was blocked by the meat and dairy industries, because they claimed it stigmatized their products.[4] The USDA had placed them under the category "eat less." Afraid of losing business, both industries lashed out at the USDA. As a result, the original 1992 pyramid was changed, despite the knowledge that these food groups should be consumed less frequently and not more.

The pyramid was updated in early 2005. Sadly, this replacement was not very different from the first. The only major difference highlighted in the newer chart was the elimination of the entire portion that contained mostly refined carbohydrates and "white foods," such as bread, pasta, and cookies. This change showed positive progress, however confused consumers complained to the USDA that the New Pyramid was not easy to understand. Another issue was that the revised chart was primarily made available via the Internet. This posed a dilemma for those who were not technologically savvy or didn't have access to the Internet. According to the U.S. Census Bureau, at the time of this printing, more than 20 percent of people in the United States still do not have access to the Internet.[5] Therefore, twenty out of every hundred people do not have access to the pyramid.

In 2011 First Lady Michelle Obama decided to take a proactive stand on health in the United States and waged a full-on nutrition war. She planted an organic garden at the White House and then pushed for the USDA to tackle the food pyramid again, hoping to make it more concise and clear.

What was the result of Michelle's hard work? The Pyramid is out, and the Plate is in. The new MyPlate (see Figure 2 on page 83) debuted to Americans in the summer of 2011. It still advises dairy as a large portion of the diet, despite Marion Nestle's recommendations in 1992. Otherwise, thankfully, the Plate is much simpler than the outdated Pyramid. The Pyramid model did not necessarily translate diet into everyday life, but the Plate actually shows you how to build a plate of food. For example, half your plate should consist of fruits and vegetables. The necessity of this format shows that, despite the changes that have been made over the past twenty years, we still have a long way to go in educating Americans on proper nutrition.

Back to Nature: Organics 101

As a consumer, the more educated you are about the foods you choose, the better your health will be. You cannot expect the food industry to be your health advocate. It is up to you to learn as much as you can about what you put into your body. The benefits you will receive in return will be bountiful health and vitality.

Rule of thumb number one when choosing foods for IBD: If your great-grandmother would not recognize it on the shelf, put the item back. I repeat: Don't think, just put it back. For instance, your great-grandmother would probably not recognize microwave popcorn, which likely contains artificial colors and flavors. She wouldn't be able to recognize a TV dinner, a pound of bologna, or a can of HI-C. She would be confused by a can of Spam or even prepackaged cookies. That's because up until about the past sixty or seventy years, we did not shop exclusively in a supermarket, as most Americans do now. Food came from farmers' markets, a bakery, and a butcher. The huge difference is that nearly everything used to be unprocessed and homemade.

Rule of thumb number two: Choose organic foods whenever possible. Until about the 1950s, produce was free of pesticides, genetically modified organisms (GMOs), herbicides, fungicides, and wax. Meat and dairy products did not contain antibiotics or growth hormones and were not irradiated (exposed to radiation in an effort to "protect" us from food poisoning—a practice that alters the nutrient content and physical properties of the plant).

Today's food supply has changed drastically. Everything Great-Grandma ate was organic, but some of what people consume now cannot even be classified as food. For example, genetically modified foods are made using desirable plant genes and cross-breeding them with other plant species. An ear of corn may contain genes from as many as three other plants. If that isn't strange enough, try this on for size: In the 2008 PBS documentary *King Korn*, filmmaker Curt Ellis shows that corn today is "Round-Up Ready" (RUR), meaning that this type of corn has been bioengineered to contain genes that are undesirable to insects. In fact, when bugs eat these plants, they die.[6] Although the practice of cross-breeding plants of the same type used to happen through the process of natural selection, today it happens in laboratories through bio-engineering.

The *International Journal of Biological Sciences* conducted a study that suggested these changes have great impacts on our health. A group of rats was fed a diet of three varieties of RUR GMO corn— namely, NK 603, MON 810, and MON 863—for a period of ninety days. Because the RUR corn contained residue from Round Up, the rats were eating corn with toxic chemicals built right into the DNA.

The study showed that the reactions varied depending on the type of GMO corn. When fed MON 810, the rats showed significant gender-related problems, meaning the male rats had different issues than the female rats. The female rats experienced unfavorable changes in blood-cell counts, adrenal issues, and changes in kidney and spleen weight. The males experienced problems with liver functions. The control group was fed non-genetically-modified corn. These rats did not experience any significant health changes.[7]

The study's results are alarming and should be a wake-up call for anyone invested in maintaining optimum health. We have only been consuming GMO corn since the seventies, so the long-term effects on humans are largely unknown. It is safe to say that if the corn kills bugs and makes rats sick, we are in a bit of trouble. Our grandparents were never exposed to GMO foods, such as high-fructose corn syrup, so who knows how future generations will be affected. Pesticides, which have been shown to cause liver, kidney, and blood diseases and cancer, create extra work for the immune system.[8] They lodge and accumulate in tissue, resulting in a weakened immune system and consequently allow other carcinogens and pathogens to filter into the body and affect our health. Organic certification is the public's assurance that products have been grown and handled according to strict procedures without persistent toxic chemical inputs. For those with IBD, avoiding GMOs, pesticides, and other assorted petrochemicals in conventional produce would be wise. Sticking to organic is your best bet.

Here are the top six reasons to eat organic foods:

1. **Pesticides have no place in our bodies.** Pesticides are poisons designed to kill living organisms and thus are harmful to humans. Unfortunately, many EPA-approved pesticides were registered long before extensive research linked these chemicals to cancer and other diseases. Buying organic produce, dairy products, and meat is a way to prevent more of these chemicals from getting into the air, water, and food supply.

2. **We have to protect our water supply.** A 2008 U.S. Geologi-

cal Society study claimed that pesticides pollute the public's primary source of drinking water for more than *half* of the country's population.[9]

3. **Organic farmers work in harmony with nature.** Three billion tons of topsoil are eroded from croplands in the United States each year, and much of this loss is due to conventional farming practices that often ignore the health of the soil.[10]

    Organic agriculture respects the balance necessary for a healthy ecosystem; wildlife is encouraged by including forage crops in rotation and by retaining fencerows, wetlands, and other natural areas. Additionally, the beneficial bacteria contained in soil, known as homeostatic soil organisms (HSOs), help us break down our foods. HSOs are not present in conventionally farmed produce, because it is sprayed with chemicals. This is a shame, because HSOs have been proven to help those with IBD.[11]

4. **Let's promote biodiversity.** Planting large plots of land with the same crop year after year tripled farm production between 1950 and 1970, but the lack of natural diversity of plant life has negatively affected soil quality.[12] For those with IBD, variety is important to ensure a wide spectrum of nutrient consumption, especially for those with food intolerance. For example, instead of just consuming Idaho russet potatoes, try red potatoes, fingerling potatoes, sweet potatoes, yams, or even purple potatoes! Each variety contains different nutritional content, allowing for a more balanced diet.

5. **Eat more vitamins and minerals.** Organic farming starts with the nourishment of the soil, which in turn produces nourishing plants. Well-balanced soil produces strong, healthy plants that have more nutrients than conventionally grown produce. Studies have overwhelmingly shown that organic produce carries as much as five times more vitamins and minerals than conventional produce.[13]

6. **Savor the flavor.** Organic produce simply tastes better. Try an organic strawberry to see what I am talking about. Conduct your own taste test with different types of produce.

Sugar and IBD

Researchers have proven that people with Crohn's disease typically eat more sugar.[14] Do you feel like you eat a significant amount of sugar? Current estimates show that the average American consumes 142 pounds of sugar each year![15] That is the equivalent of seventy-one two-pound boxes per year per person. This figure is also misleading, because this statistic excludes people who avoid sugar or cannot eat sugar. Thus, some Americans actually eat *more* than 142 pounds annually.

If you have Crohn's disease, which is an inflammatory condition, it would be wise to consider reducing or eliminating sugar from your diet because it is considered an inflammatory food. This is often easier said than done, especially if you are accustomed to consuming moderate to high amounts of the sweet stuff.

Sugar is a tough habit to quit. It is sweet, seductive, and *sneaky*. Sugar is in everything from cookies to baby food. It is the reason strawberry cheesecake tantalizes your taste buds and teases your palate. It is the reason you love ice cream and have warm fuzzy memories of the corner candy store as a kid. The downside of consuming all that sugar? Your great-grandmother warned you about sugar rotting your teeth, but even your wise old granny wasn't prepared for the health crisis brought on by the sugar-laden standard American diet today.

Nutrition experts consider sugar to be a massive contributor to the current digestive disease epidemic in the United States. Research has demonstrated that high sugar and carbohydrate intake significantly contributes to the development of IBD. Although researchers did not differentiate between Crohn's disease and ulcerative colitis, both di- and monosaccharide consumption increased the risk of developing IBD in general.[16] Sucrose was consistently associated with increased risk for IBD, and the trend was statistically significant in patients with Crohn's disease. Patients with IBD had a significantly lower intake of fruit, fiber, and vegetables. (It should be noted that although fruit contains the natural sugar fructose, it doesn't produce the same issues for those with IBD that refined sugars do.)

Another study confirmed a higher intake of total carbohydrates, starch, and refined sugars in 104 patients prior to diagnosis of Crohn's disease.[17] A population-based, case-controlled Swedish study examining 152 Crohn's disease cases found a significant 3.4-fold increase in relative risk for developing Crohn's disease when consuming fast food two to three times weekly.[18] Fast food is loaded with sugar, so these results make sense.

Top wellness gurus, such as Dr. Joseph Mercola and Marion Nestle, attribute this level of consumption to ignorance and insufficient labeling laws. The average person does not know that sugar can also be called sucrose, fructose, dextrose, maltose, sorbitol, or maltitol—just to name a few. Our sneaky friend sugar has found its way into our bodies via everything from super-refined high-fructose corn syrup to organic evaporated cane juice, which is mistakenly thought to be "healthy." There is no place to hide from it. Sugar is in your face every day.

The best way to avoid the sweet stuff is to become knowledgeable and conscious of your dietary habits. Learn how to look for sugars, including alternative names the government allows companies to call it, ultimately confusing the average consumer. And let's face it: You can't totally deprive yourself. So how can you get plenty of sweetness in life without worrying about the negative health implications? Start by following my "Top Five Tips for Beating a Sugar Addiction."

Top Five Tips for Beating a Sugar Addiction

The following little tricks will help you say good-bye to the white (and also the brown) stuff:

1. Drink more water.

Are you thirsty? In most cases, you are craving sugar because you are dehydrated. Your body does not send a signal alerting you to thirst until you are actually on the brink of dehydration. The next time you are craving a chocolate-covered pretzel, ask yourself when you last had water. If you have had fewer than the eight daily-recommended servings, try drinking a glass or two and see how you feel. Has the craving dissipated? This is a great trick.

2. Eat more sweet fruits and vegetables.

Imagine you were alive 500 years ago. A grocery store would be foreign to you. A candy bar would be a rare commodity, if it even existed. Thus, if you craved something sweet, you wouldn't be thinking of a Boston cream doughnut but rather an apple or a sweet potato. A craving for sweets could indicate a lack of fruits and vegetables. Try some sweet veggies, such as corn, sweet potatoes, spaghetti squash, carrots, parsnips, pumpkin, onions, and tomatoes. An apple, banana, or grapes all contain higher amounts of fructose, the naturally occurring sugar in fruit.

3. Avoid the white diet.

Evaluate your intake of white foods, such as cookies, bread, cupcakes, and pretzels. These foods are refined carbohydrates, meaning they are "empty" calories that contain virtually zero nutritional content. When you eat foods that are highly processed and void of nutritional value, you are doing the body a disservice and adding to your sugar cravings. These simple carbohydrates break down very quickly in the body, causing your blood sugar levels to rise rapidly and then to decline. When this happens, you will need to eat more frequently to balance your blood sugar. This cycle can then cause cravings for more of these types of junk foods. Your best bet is to avoid them and replace them with whole grains.

4. Eat more whole grains.

Some people eat sugar because they think it will give them an energy boost. And yes, there is truth to that, but this boost is temporary and causes your kidneys and pancreas to work overtime to produce insulin for processing the sugar. How do you gain long-lasting energy *and* avoid stressing your organs? Eat complex carbohydrates, such as brown rice, millet, quinoa, amaranth, buckwheat, corn, wheat, rye, barley, oats, fruits, and vegetables. These foods contain natural sugars in addition to essential vitamins, minerals, and amino acids. These nutrients allow you to eat a small amount of food and become full faster and for longer time periods, reducing the need for excess sugar in the diet.

5. Try natural sweeteners.

Some great new sweeteners are actually healthy for you. Be adventurous the next time you are in the store and try one out. Agave nectar is an excellent natural liquid sweetener that comes from a cactus plant.

It is low on the glycemic index and therefore safe for diabetics. Agave is also 1.4 times sweeter than regular sugar, so it will satisfy your sweet tooth. Raw honey, molasses, and real maple syrup are all oldies but goodies. Any of these natural sweeteners contain an array of vitamins, with some kinds of molasses being the powerhouse, as they can contain a perfect blend of magnesium, potassium, phosphorus, and iron. Stevia is another wonderful sweetener that has recently become popular. It comes from the leaves of the stevia plant and is sold under the brand name Truvia.

. . . .

As you become more mindful of your sugar intake, you may realize you were eating way too much of the stuff. When you read labels, watch out for the words "corn syrup," "high-fructose corn syrup," "evaporated cane juice," "sucrose," "dextrose," "maltose," and "fructose," all of which are different names for sugar.

After a month of following these tips, make a note of the positive changes you've made and keep moving forward. Removing or reducing sugar from the diet is meant to be a gradual process, but it can yield results for a lifetime. By adding new foods, you'll eventually acquire a taste for healthier food instead. These tried and true suggestions really work if you make the effort.

Quiz Are You a Sugar Junkie?

✓ What role does sugar play in your life? Take this quiz to determine whether sugar consumption is an issue you want to work on. Follow the suggestions at the end of the test to find steps to kick the sugar habit.

1. **What is your breakfast like?**
    A. eggs and toast with fruit
    B. brown rice pudding with coconut milk, carrots, raisins, and walnuts
    C. doughnuts with coffee

2. **When you are at a party, which selection is most appetizing for you?**
    A. the yummy salad and veggie appetizers
    B. hello, the birthday cake, of course!
    C. chips and dip

3. **What is your ideal snack?**
   A. a salty, warm, jumbo pretzel
   B. fruit
   C. nachos with fresh salsa, avocado, and shredded cheddar

4. **When you have coffee or tea, how many sugars/honey servings do you use?**
   A. None, I like it plain.
   B. One or two are fine for me.
   C. One or two are not going to cut it!

5. **You're at the office, restless before an upcoming meeting. You want to be focused during the meeting, so you decide you need to refuel. In the cafeteria, what do you choose?**
   A. a grilled vegetable wrap with soup
   B. a large coffee and a candy bar
   C. a yogurt and granola parfait

6. **How often do you drink soda, eat candy, or eat junk foods?**
   A. rarely or never
   B. several times a week
   C. daily

7. **When at the movies, what is your favorite snack?**
   A. Skittles
   B. dark-chocolate-covered Raisinets
   C. popcorn

8. **When eating out, which would be your favorite appetizer?**
   A. chips with spinach artichoke dip
   B. breadsticks with marinara sauce
   C. coconut shrimp with pineapple marmalade

9. **How do you feel about your weight?**
   A. I am right on target or would like to gain a few pounds.
   B. I could lose a few pounds.
   C. I miss my skinny jeans, because I have moved up a few sizes.

10. **Would you be mad if someone took the sugar out of your iced tea or coffee?**
    A. Yes, that would take some getting used to.
    B. There is no way I would drink my beverages unsweetened!
    C. No, that really wouldn't bother me.

Answer Key:

Here are the point levels for each answer. Circle the point value that corresponds to how your answered each question, and then write your total in the space provided.

QUESTION	ANSWER A	ANSWER B	ANSWER C
1	2	1	3
2	1	2	2
3	3	2	1
4	1	2	3
5	1	3	2
6	1	2	3
7	2	2	1
8	2	3	1
9	1	2	3
10	2	3	1

My total score: _____

Score 0–10—Low Priority

Sugar does not really excite you. Based on the results of this quiz, you do not consume a significant amount of sugar. With a score as low as this, it could be safe to say that you are not a sugar junkie. Bravo! Continue to be mindful of your sugar consumption. You may benefit from journaling when you do have sweet stuff to see how it affects your IBD. It wouldn't hurt to check out some of the natural sweeteners below. These are healthier for you than table sugar, which can contribute to more than 120 different health concerns.[19]

Score 11–20—Medium Priority

Sugar shows up in your diet in several places. This can be concerning, because it may very well be contributing to your IBD symptoms. To beat your sugar addiction, evaluate the following lifestyle factors:

Dehydration—When you are dehydrated, instead of sending a signal to alert you to drink, many times the brain will trigger signals for your sweet cravings. Try drinking a glass of water prior to binging on a sugary snack and see how you feel.

Lack of sweet fruits and vegetables—Most people think cravings are bad; however, some let you know which vitamins and minerals your body needs. If you consistently desire sweet foods, evaluate your intake of fruits and veggies. Perhaps you are not getting the recommended servings per day, and your body is actually requesting nutrients naturally occurring in these foods.

Reduce or eliminate caffeine intake—Caffeine can produce blood-sugar swings, causing you to crave sugar to temporarily boost your energy levels. Limit your caffeine consumption as much as possible.

Stress levels—Sometimes stress can cause certain food cravings. Review the Wheel of Digestive Health on page 35 to evaluate the areas of your life that are causing anxiety. Make a plan to work on these areas using the goal sheets in Chapter 1. See how your sugar intake evolves after you make these lifestyle changes.

Evaluate meat intake in your diet—The body is always looking to achieve balance. Thus eating a diet with excessive amounts of animal protein may make you crave sugar. Pay attention to your meat intake and journal your sugar cravings after consuming them.[20]

Score 21–30—High Priority

Sugar plays a large role in your life. Your consumption of it is on the high side, and you should pay close attention to it. Aside from aggravating IBD symptoms, sugar can also contribute to diabetes, cancer, hypoglycemia, multiple sclerosis, lupus, arthritis, weakened immune functioning, issues with magnesium and calcium absorption, depression, Alzheimer's disease, headaches, migraines, and even heart disease.[21]

Follow the aforementioned instructions for dealing with sugar cravings, including the tips in the sections for low- and medium-priority scores. Take advantage of the natural sweeteners listed on pages 92 and 93 to satisfy your sweet tooth. You can also check out the recipe section to look for some healthier alternatives.

One extra tip: Anytime you are craving a treat, allow yourself to indulge only if you make the item from scratch. This approach serves two purposes. One, you know exactly what is in the food. When you buy something packaged, it likely contains artificial ingredients, such as high-fructose corn syrup, flavors, or coloring, whereas making your sweets at home allows you to control the quality of ingredients. Two, the less easy access you have to sweets, the less likely you are to overindulge. For example, if you are craving cake and have to bake it yourself, would you normally take the time to do this? Most times, I find people would not.

Caffeine Consumption and IBD

Caffeine is one common factor in the standard American diet that stands out when it comes to complicating Crohn's and colitis. Drinking coffee is one of the most challenging dietary habits to change because it is addictive and so entrenched in our culture.[22] For many, a cup of coffee is synonymous to waking up in the morning, and its consumption is considered completely routine. Caffeine withdrawal can produce a whole host of side effects, including headaches, vomiting, nausea, and loose stools.[23] The following are negative effects caffeine can cause when introduced to the intestinal tract.

Coffee Elevates Stress Hormones, Affecting the Adrenal Glands and Digestive Tract

Caffeine increases the body's production of stress hormones, including cortisol, epinephrine (adrenaline), and norepinephrine.[24] Because caffeine causes increased heart rate and blood pressure, drinking it puts your digestive system in a state of emergency. In an effort to purge it from the body, blood is diverted from the digestive system causing indigestion. If that wasn't enough, the brain then blocks oxygen from the extremities in an effort to "protect" them, and the immune system becomes depressed. This reaction can eventually cause your body to become more susceptible to infections and can slow down healing time.

Coffee Increases Bowel Movements

Because caffeine stimulates the digestive tract to overactivity, coffee and excessive bowel movements can go together. For those of you who spend a considerable amount of time in the bathroom already, this is probably not welcome news. As quickly as four minutes after consumption, coffee produces a laxative effect and stimulates recto-sigmoid motor activity. Even miniscule doses of coffee can have this negative effect or produce loose stool. Studies have shown that even decaf has a similar stimulant effect on the GI tract.[25]

Coffee Has a Negative Impact on GABA Metabolism

GABA (gamma-aminobutyric acid) is a neurotransmitter produced by the brain and digestive tract that is responsible for mood and stress management. It has been known to have a calming effect on the GI tract. *Molecular Pharmacology* published a study showing caffeine has been found to interfere with the binding of GABA to GABA receptors.[26] This does not allow the GABA to properly soothe the digestive tract. Did you ever drink coffee and then feel anxious? Pay attention to how you feel the next time you enjoy a cup. You may be surprised that caffeine does not really give you the effect you want.

Coffee Can Cause a pH Imbalance

Just like the pool in your backyard needs to be kept at the proper pH, your body also requires an appropriate balance between acid and alkaline foods to maintain optimum health. If your system becomes overly acidic or alkaline it can cause ill health effects. (I go into specific details about pH and IBD in Chapter 4.) For now, just understand that coffee is highly acidic and can stimulate the hypersecretion of gastric acids. Decaf also fails to be healthier, as research has shown that it actually causes a greater acidity level than its caffeinated counterparts.[27]

Coffee Decreases Magnesium Absorption

Caffeine also affects the way your body metabolizes magnesium—an essential mineral if you have IBD. It is primarily known for its role in maintaining bowel regularity, among three hundred other bodily functions. Magnesium not only promotes bowel regularity but it also can produce a laxative effect that resolves constipation. Additionally, magnesium has been found to be crucial in wound healing, which is significant for patients with IBD, as it affects how the intestinal lining heals.[28]

Tips for Kicking the Caffeine Habit

If you have IBD, it is best to avoid caffeine if you do not already consume it. If you partake in the addiction on a regular basis, you may have tried to quit unsuccessfully. Here are some tips for reducing your caffeine-withdrawal symptoms to make the process easier.

Gradually decrease coffee consumption by a quarter cup daily each week. For example, if you normally drink 2 cups of coffee a day, the first week you would drink 1¾ cups, the second week 1½ cups, the third week 1¼ cups, and the fourth week you would be down to 1 cup a day. Keep up this process until you are coffee free.

Try drinking tea instead. You can swap out healthier alternatives like green tea, chamomile, pau d'arco, or anything else that you happen to like. Although green, black, and white teas still contain caffeine, they contain considerably less than coffee (40 mg caffeine per cup in green tea versus 120 mg per cup in coffee). The benefits of drinking these teas generally outweigh the risks, because they also contain ECGC, a very potent antioxidant.

Try Teeccino, the herbal coffee supplement. Teeccino is a product available for those who like the taste of coffee but don't want the negative side effects. It is made from carob, barley, almond, figs, and dates. Teeccino offers excellent health benefits, including promoting alkalinity in the body which is great for IBD sufferers whose systems tend to be overly acidic. This beverage is also a significant source of potassium. Give it a try and see what you think! It is a favorite among my clients, so I recommend all of the time. You can order it at http://www.teeccino.com.

Chapter 4

. . . .

Soothing Foods for the Intestines

Chapter 3 discussed foods that are unsupportive of digestion. This chapter introduces dietary plans and foods that can help soothe your intestinal tract and improve your digestion. Because there is no one right way of eating for everybody, evaluate the information provided in each section. You can try out some of the theories and see which things work best for you.

Michael's Story

Michael came to see me after being diagnosed with celiac disease. He was in his late thirties and reported experiencing brain fog, acne, and psoriasis. He was overweight, and, despite being gluten-free for six months, he was still having digestive symptoms, such as gas, bloating, and constipation. This client had been tested by his doctor for iron deficiency and was also anemic.

Because Michael had had such terrible inflammation in his gut for such a long time prior to his diagnosis, he really needed an anti-inflammatory diet to help him heal. He also needed specific amino acids to mend the lining of the intestines.

Michael admitted to being a sugar addict. This was the worst thing for Michael, because sugar can cause a great deal of inflammation. I recommended that Michael consume anti-inflammatory foods, such as pineapple, coconut, olive, walnut, avocado, and flax oils, and foods that are soothing for indigestion, such as millet. For his sugar fix, I recommended that Michael try frozen bananas or make a fruit purée smoothie and freeze it as an ice pop. We worked diligently to add more of these healing foods to his diet while eliminating the unhealthy foods.

As his sugar consumption dwindled, so did the amount of acne he had. This change motivated him to be even more particular about his diet. Michael testified he had gone from hiding his face to playfully flaunting it. But more meaningfully, his digestion improved as the amino acids assisted in the repair of his stomach lining and his diet remained based on whole foods rather than junk foods. He learned how to nourish his body and pay attention to its many signals. After studying for an exam, Michael reported his ability to concentrate had improved drastically, and he found it wonderfully strange to know that he didn't have to work as hard at math, normally his worst subject.

 The Pumped-Up Piña Colada Smoothie on page 167 would double as an excellent ice pop and is one of Michael's favorites. The coconut milk and the bromelain in the pineapple are both anti-inflammatory and soothing to the intestines.

Anti-Inflammatory Foods

Inflammation can be caused by many things, including environmental factors and foods. Everyone's body is different. As discussed in Chapter 2, certain foods produce an inflammatory effect in some individuals with food intolerance. However, other items can cause inflammation in virtually all humans. These include *sugar, processed foods, trans fats, hydrogenated oils, smoked meats containing nitrates, preservatives, and artificial colorings and flavorings.*[1] To maintain intestinal health, decrease your consumption of inflammatory or reactive foods and increase your intake of healthier alternatives.

This chart below is adapted from one originally created by Dr. Andrew Weil. I was quite fortunate to study under this renowned physician in the alternative health-care field. It serves as an excellent guideline for those with IBD, as it provides a clear idea of foods that can decrease inflammation. These foods are recommended for daily consumption but will also soothe flare-ups in most cases.

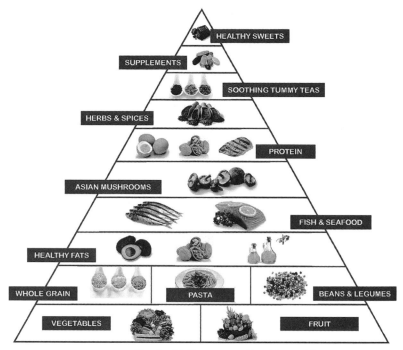

FIGURE 3. The Anti-inflammatory Food Pyramid

Fruits and Vegetables

Not surprisingly, fruits and vegetables are now considered the least-consumed foods in the standard American diet, although they are arguably the most important for improving health. Can you guess what is the number-one consumed veggie is? Potatoes, in the infamous form of French fries. The runner-up is tomatoes, in the form of high-fructose corn syrup–based ketchup.[2] Because fast food is so accessible and inexpensive, it is no wonder that produce has escaped our modern diet. The number-one dilemma my clients stress about is lack of time, with the majority claiming they are too busy to cook. I can appreciate a busy lifestyle; however, raw vegetables and fruits can be readily accessible if you know where to look and are willing to do a little preparation.

In as little as ten minutes, you can prepare a snack of some carrot sticks with hummus or celery with peanut butter. Grabbing an apple or banana in the morning as you are leaving the house is simple, quick, and an excellent healthy habit to develop. It is crucial for good digestion to get enough fiber, minerals, vitamins, phytochemicals, phytonutrients, enzymes, and beneficial bacteria that only plant-based foods can provide. In my experience, a diet without fiber-filled fruits and vegetables is *always a disaster* for the gut. When I look at a client's health history and see these staples are missing, what does that leave the individual with? The answer is mostly meat, refined grains, and processed fast foods. This poses its own problem, as these convenience foods are made with unhealthy omega-6 fatty acids and lack healthy omega-3 fatty acids. This type of diet is a recipe for inflammation that can contribute to Crohn's disease and colitis, as noted in *New Medicine: The Complete Family Health Guide.*[3]

And if that doesn't convince you that you *must* eat your veggies, just rely on common sense. We have been consuming vegetables and fruits since the beginning of time, but we were *not* pulling through drive-through windows and eating fried foods with highly refined sugars until about the 1950s. Keep a food diary for a week, and you may be shocked at the lack of fruits and veggies in your diet. Don't fret over the results, but embrace the simple changes you should make (as noted above) to get on the right track.

The Top Eight Fruits and Veggies to Consume When You Have a Flare-Up

I have had many clients come in to my office with a flare-up and tell me they are afraid to eat vegetables and fruits for fear that doing so will make their flare-up worse. Actually, and to the contrary, it is helpful to add fresh, organic, steamed fruits and vegetables to your diet as long as your doctor does not have you on bowel rest. They are chock full of nutrition that can help you alleviate your symptoms, Just make sure you chew them very well.

1. Leafy, Green Vegetables

We know the number-one veggie is a potato, so what is the number-one type of food missing from the average American's diet? Dark, green, leafy vegetables. It is often evident to me that these are badly needed when clients inquire what the following look like, because they are completely foreign to many Americans. These include kale, collard greens, mustard greens, watercress, arugula, romaine, broccoli, broccoli rabe, and Swiss chard. Dark green vegetables provide many essential phytochemicals and nutrients, such as vitamins A, D, and C, and minerals, like potassium, magnesium, and phosphorus.

Green "leafies" are also important for eliminating depression and strengthening the lungs, kidneys, and adrenal glands. Most important for those with IBD, leafy greens have been known to promote healthy intestinal flora, which in turn helps the immune system.[4] If you cannot tolerate the greens in their raw form, you can always lightly steam them to make them more digestible. Additionally, you may want to remove the stems from kale and Swiss chard. Although they are edible, they are difficult to break down and are best avoided by those with IBD.

You can also juice leafy green vegetables or buy smoothie drinks that contain them, such as Naked Green Machine, which contains puréed fruit to sweeten the flavor. I love being able to add these types of drinks to my diet, especially for days when I'm on the run and notice I haven't gotten my green vegetable fix. It's almost like an insurance policy, making sure I get the nutrition I need with almost no effort.

2. Coconut Milk or Water

Coconut milk is known to have anti-inflammatory properties, because it contains omega-3 long-chain fatty acids. Coconut water is excellent, especially in cases of dehydration. It contains more electrolytes than Gatorade and a considerable amount of potassium. Potassium is one of the first minerals to become depleted when you have become dehydrated. Lauric acid in coconut oil has also been found to have antimicrobial factors, meaning it can fight off bad bacteria and viruses. The caprylic acid in coconut oil is effective for treating excessive yeast overgrowth in the body, which can complicate symptoms for those with IBD.[5] If you are having a flare-up, coconut milk or water should definitely be a staple in your diet.

3. Puréed Fruits and Vegetables

When you are having a flare-up, foods can be difficult to break down. A great alternative to eating your daily diet is to go back to basics for a while. Try some organic baby food, or purée your own combinations.

Make sure you choose fruits and vegetables high in vitamins B and C from the yellow and orange food groups, such as bananas, oranges, and sweet potatoes, because they are essential to replenishing your energy levels and antioxidants when you lose too much fluid. A nurse recommended this to me while I had a flare-up years ago, and now I suggest it to clients all the time. Read *Super Baby Foods*, by Ruth Yaron, for some interesting and tasty purée combinations.

 Turn leftover fruits and veggies into puréed smoothies and juices. Smoothies and juices are highly recommended, because they provide an excellent way to receive highly absorbable nutrition. This is vital when you have a flare-up or are on bowel rest. Make your own or try something freshly juiced from the health-food store. You can find tons of recipes on various websites and, of course, check out those featured in this book's recipe section.

4. Shiitake and Maitake Mushrooms

Shiitake and maitake mushrooms help boost the immune system.[6] They can be included in stir-fries and casseroles and make a welcome addition to any meal.

5. Pineapple

Pineapples contain the enzyme bromelain, which increases your digestive ability and even destroys intestinal worms. This fruit is also known for its ability to eradicate diarrhea and indigestion.[7]

6. Papaya

Papayas are a super food for those with IBD. Its fantastic abilities include strengthening the abdominal muscles, treating indigestion, clearing excessive mucus (especially helpful for those with food intolerance), and serving as a digestive aid. Additionally, the seeds of underripe papayas contain the enzyme bromelain.[8]

7. Cabbage

Cabbage is wonderful for promoting intestinal health, especially when it is fermented. Raw sauerkraut is the best form, as it provides beneficial enzymes making it easier to metabolize.[9] Cabbage is also good for lubricating the intestines and serves as a digestive aid. It is also helpful in strengthening the stomach and clearing up constipation. It is great for ulcers and eradicating digestive worms.[10]

8. Celery

Celery is known for its beneficial properties in aiding digestion and for its benefits to the stomach.[11] Celery may be eaten raw or juiced, if better tolerated. A delicious mix to try is celery, kale, and apple.

Whole Grains

Some people are not really sure what whole grains actually are. Advertising has taught us that staple breakfast cereals are whole grains, when actually they are broken down, processed versions of the real thing. Real whole grains are essentially whole. They still have their nutritional integrity intact and exist in their unrefined, natural state. Foods contained in the grain family are amaranth, barley, buckwheat, corn, millet, oats, quinoa, rye, teff, and wheat. I will focus on three here that are particularly helpful during flare-ups.

Brown Rice

Brown rice is an excellent food to have on hand, especially for flare-ups. Part of the BRAT diet (bananas, rice, apples, and toast) normally prescribed to alleviate chronic diarrhea, brown rice is an effective binding agent that helps counter diarrhea, yet it also contains fiber, allowing you to comfortably pass bowel movements. This grain can be prepared as a porridge, as detailed in the recipe section of this book. It also contains a significant amount of water, so it rehydrates the cells.[12]

Buckwheat

Contrary to its name, buckwheat, also known as kasha, is part of the rhubarb family of plants and does not actually contain any wheat. You may already have eaten buckwheat in its noodle form, as soba. Beware of soba noodles when eating out, as many manufacturers cut the buckwheat flour with the cheaper wheat flour, causing problems for those with gluten and wheat issues.

Buckwheat is an ideal food for endurance, and it is also one of only two grains that contain all eight essential amino acids, making it a complete protein. High in vitamins B and E, buckwheat is fantastic for your skin, metabolism, memory, concentration, and more.

Millet

Gluten-free and easy to digest, millet is ideal for those with IBD. This grain contains iron; vitamins B-1, B-2, and B-3; phosphorous; magnesium; and zinc. B vitamins are important for intestinal contractions and allow waste materials to pass through the intestines. Millet eases constipation, but it is also binding if you have diarrhea. These properties make millet a super food for those with IBD. For maximum digestibility, when preparing millet, rinse it in cold water first. For each cup of the grain, add four cups of water. It will turn out slightly mushy, but this consistency is best for absorption when you have a flare-up or are showing IBD symptoms. Add some fruit juice for extra flavor.

Quinoa

Quinoa is another easy-to-digest, gluten-free grain. It has been touted by Native-American Indians for centuries for its nutritional properties. Like buckwheat, it contains all eight essential amino acids, making it a complete protein. Quinoa contains a host of vitamins and minerals, including calcium and iron. You can prepare this grain in a number of ways, such as a replacement for rice with stir-fries. Additionally, you can make it the same way that you prepare millet.

Essential Fatty Acids

Coconut oil, which is derived from fruit, contains essential omega-3 fatty acids, which are responsible for building healthy brain cells, controlling inflammation in the intestines, and protecting the heart.[13] Most people today do not get enough omega-3s.

You can find healthy fats in the following foods:

- avocados
- chia seeds
- flaxseed
- grass-fed organic beef

- herring
- mackerel
- salmon
- sardines

- sesame seeds
- tuna
- walnuts

These are very important foods if you have IBD, as they can help repair the damage in your gut. Try to consume omega-3s at least once or twice per day. If you don't remember to eat these foods, you can always review the recommended supplements in Chapter 5, specifically fish and flaxseed oils.

IBD and the Vegetarian/Vegan Diet

If you have cut meat from your diet for ethical or health purposes, good for you! A vegetarian diet is free of meat and poultry and generally consists of proteins from foods such as dairy, beans, nuts, seeds, and eggs. People who do not eat meat but do consume fish are called pescetarians. A vegan diet is more restricted, eliminating any food that is derived from an animal, including honey, fish, dairy, and eggs. Embarking on a limited diet can be a challenge, but being a vegetarian can work well for those with IBD. As shown in the earlier discussion of the Loma Linda, California, blue zone (see page 23), this type of diet can offer a plethora of health benefits, but vegetarians must be aware of a few things to ensure they remain in the best health.

Rule #1 for IBD Vegetarians/Vegans: Have Your Vitamin Levels Checked

Of all the vitamin deficiencies I see in my practice and at my corporate job, nearly all IBD or "digestively" challenged cases share one particular issue: lack of B-vitamin absorption and production. This is due to the specific way these vitamins are absorbed through intrinsic and extrinsic factors in the intestines (please see page 125 for more information). If your intestines are inflamed, you can bet you're not absorbing sufficient B vitamins that prevent such ailments as vomiting, nausea, fatigue, and even depression, anxiety, and weight gain.[14] B vitamins also fuel peristaltic contractions in the intestines, which are the muscle contractions responsible for passing waste through the gut. Without them, you would not have proper bowel movements and you will likely suffer from constipation. Why is this an issue for vegetarians, and even more so for vegans? Most B vitamins come from animal sources, so eat plenty of whole or cracked grains that are high in this vitamin, including brown rice, millet, buckwheat, and quinoa. You will also want to supplement your diet with vitamin B-12, preferably sublingual (under the tongue) because its high absorbability is best for those with compromised digestion.

Rule #2 for IBD Vegetarians/Vegans: Get Enough Protein

One frequent argument that vegetarians and vegans endure from nonvegetarians is the ominous protein debate. Proteins are the building blocks of amino acids, which are crucial to emotional and physical well-being. Protein is required for the regulation of the organs in the body, cell production, and growth. Some experts recommend vegetarian diets, including Michio Kushi, founder of the macrobiotic diet and author of *The Macrobiotic Way*. Macrobiotics focus on eating fruits; vegetables; whole grains; healthy fats, such as walnuts and avocados; and fermented foods, such as miso and umeboshi plum vinegar. Other experts, such as Dr. Robert Atkins, founder of the namesake diet, completely disagree. Most will remember the Atkins Diet, which phased out somewhat after the initial fad in early 2000. Atkins showed promising research on the benefits of eating high quantities of protein via meat and fewer carbohydrates. My position on protein is that as long as you get your daily protein requirements and listen to your body, you should be fine. The ratios below can be used by vegetarians, vegans, and meat eaters alike to calculate daily protein-intake requirements. If you are doing well, you can use the 0.8 ratio. If you just had a flare-up or are recovering from surgery, you will want more protein, so use 1.8. In the example below, an individual weighing 130 pounds who was recently hospitalized for an obstruction should follow the 0.8 ratio, so this person would need about 106.23 grams of protein daily.

▍How to Calculate Daily Protein Requirements

FIRST:	SECOND:
To get your weight in kg, divide your weight in pounds by 2.2	To see how many grams of protein you should eat in a day, multiply your weight in kg by 0.8–1.8 gm/kg, depending on your protein needs*
Example: 130 lbs ÷ 2.2 = 59.09 weight in kg	59.09 × 1.8 gm/kg = 106.23 protein grams daily
Calculate your daily protein requirement in the space below: _____ lbs ÷ 2.2 = _____ kg; _____ kg × 1.8 gm/kg = _____ gm protein daily	

* Use the ratio of 0.8 for times when you are not flaring up and are relatively healthy. If you are recovering from a flare-up or surgery or have a heavy workout routine, your protein requirements will be higher, so you can use the 1.8 ratio.

Signs of inadequate protein intake include slow wound healing, hair loss, loss of muscle tone, anemia, skin inflammation, feeling "spacey or jittery," or excessive sugar cravings.

Vegetarians and especially vegans would greatly benefit from incorporating complete protein grains as quinoa or buckwheat, which are just about the only plant-based foods that contain all eight amino acids. These grains are quite versatile and can be served as a breakfast porridge or side dish. Enjoy the quinoa and buckwheat suggestion in the recipe section, or try experimenting on your own. If you are unable to tolerate grains, it is essential to check your amino-acid levels to determine whether you are breaking down proteins correctly. Because amino acids are most frequently found in animal-based foods, it would be a good idea to ensure you're receiving adequate amino acids. This is especially important if you are vegan and have no alternative source of animal foods.

The short story here is that what is right for one vegetarian with IBD may not be right for the next. If you have certain conditions, such as candida, which can coexist with IBD, a vegetarian or vegan diet may not be appropriate for you because animal proteins can be helpful in starving fungal overgrowth. Millet is an antifungal that does have substantial protein content, which makes it a perfect anti-candida food. As you can see, the vegetarian and vegan options can get a tad confusing, so seek out a professional's advice if you are unsure which foods would be appropriate for your digestion.

Put It All Together

If you include these foods in your diet, you should see significant improvements in your digestion over a short period of time. Check out the recipes and resources in this book if you need some creative inspiration on how to prepare these items or information on where to find them.

Here is a sample menu showing how to incorporate these foods into your diet:

Anti-Inflammatory Diet Menu

Free of dairy, gluten, and eggs

	BREAKFAST	LUNCH	DINNER
Monday	• 2 slices Enjoy Life Bread toast with cashew butter with banana • ½ cup red pepper slices	• 1 cup vegetable soup • Arugula salad with tomato, corn, turkey bacon, and radicchio • 3 tablespoons with oil and vinegar	• Grilled salmon • 1 cup brown rice • Vegetable stir-fry with sesame oil
Tuesday	• So Delicious Coconut Yogurt Parfait with granola, strawberries, and blueberries • Top with 2 tablespoons flaxseed	• Salad with romaine lettuce, turkey, carrots, edamame, and radishes • Top with sesame dressing • 1 serving coconut water	• Baked chicken with 1 cup quinoa • Steamed cauliflower with sea salt and pepper • Baked bananas with shredded coconut

(cont'd.)

▋ Anti-Inflammatory Diet Menu (cont'd.)

	BREAKFAST	LUNCH	DINNER
Wednesday	• 1 cup gluten-free oatmeal with walnuts, raisins, and shredded carrots with vanilla or chocolate rice milk • ½ cantaloupe	• Allergen-free pita with grilled zucchini, eggplant, and squash • Top with hummus • Serve with organic corn chips and salsa verde	• Brown rice pasta with plain tomato sauce • Small salad of baby greens, pecans, and cherries with cherry balsamic vinaigrette
Thursday	• Sweet Potato Pancakes (see recipe on page 147) with warm apple compote • Top with maple syrup and flaxseed	• Grilled organic chicken breast with pineapple slices • Green beans • Fermented raw sauerkraut	• Organic grass-fed steak with onions and garlic • Asparagus • Baked potato • Papaya slices
Friday	• Juice of celery, apple, Swiss chard • 1 cup cooked millet, sweetened with apple juice • Raw walnuts	• Tuna tacos • Top with lettuce, tomatoes, avocados, black beans, taco seasoning and sauce, etc.	• 1 slice cheeseless pizza with roasted kale, onions, and shiitake mushrooms • Mixed baby greens with avocado and roasted red peppers • Red-wine vinaigrette
Saturday	• Brown Rice Pudding (see recipe on page 245) • ½ cup brown rice • Coconut milk • Dried cranberries, almonds, flaxseed, and maple syrup	• Baked adzuki beans • Sweet potato • Cucumber salad • 1 serving coconut water	• Tuna and vegetables (bamboo shoots, mushrooms, zucchini) over brown rice • Watermelon slices • 1 serving coconut water
Sunday	• Whole-grain cereal* with almond milk • Flaxseed • Fruit salad	• Allergen-free pita bread with grilled mackerel, millet, salsa, scallions, and avocado	• Black bean and vegetable (spinach, carrots, celery) stir-fry over quinoa

* I suggest using Erewhon Brown Rice Dream

Healthy Anti-Inflammatory Lunch Ideas for Those on the Go

The following are some quick lunch ideas:

Monday's Lunch

- grilled chicken or vegetable fajita (in a brown-rice wrap)
- dried fruit and nut mix or a dried fruit and nut bar (for example, Lara Bar, apple pie)
- brown-rice pudding
- one serving soymilk, rice milk, or coconut milk
- gluten-free pretzels with guacamole or salsa

Tuesday's Lunch

- organic avocado mashed with Simply Organic Guacamole dressing seasoning and roasted red pepper on gluten-free corn bread
- apple slices with almond butter
- organic soy string cheese stick
- sparkling water or juice
- organic popcorn

Wednesday's Lunch

- tuna and veggies with brown rice crackers
- organic seasonal fruit and veggies (try frozen grapes or bananas)
- brown rice pasta salad
- single serve coconut water (Harvest Bay is my favorite)
- Lara Bar, such as tropical flavor

Thursday's Lunch

- organic garden vegetable and rice soup (Whole Foods 365 brand)
- celery rib with cashew butter and raisins

- baked rice pita or tortilla chips with salsa or guacamole
- Naked or Odwalla fruit smoothie
- organic fruit leather or fruit bars (no sugar added)

Friday's Lunch

- homemade vegetable soup in a thermos
- side salad with romaine, avocados, scallions, honey ginger dressing
- Enjoy Life crackers with strawberry jelly
- bottled water with lemon and lime
- natural potato chips

Chapter 5

Establishing a Supplement Regime for Inflammatory Bowel Disease

The focus of this book has been on eating to cater to food sensitivities with the goal of remaining symptom free. This chapter combines that information with a digestive wellness plan that includes specific supplement recommendations.

The supplements below are first generalized for everyone and then go into specifics to help you determine your special needs. As always, you should consult with your doctor or a nutritionist prior to embarking on any health plan.

Daphne's Story

Daphne was a referral from an amazing physician's assistant (PA) at my practice. My PA warned me that I would be taking on a tough case and ran through the laundry list of health problems challenging this client. Seemingly plagued with everything from diarrhea to depression, Daphne appeared to be diagnosed with every ailment in the book. She did not have IBD but had been formerly diagnosed with IBS. Her worst digestive complaint was urgency. She no longer could hold her bowels and had resorted to wearing a diaper. It was very frustrating for Daphne, as her lack of control had essentially rendered her disabled.

Despite her obvious plight, Daphne was very lucky, as her husband was very supportive and attended nearly every appointment. At one session in particular, he showed up with a shopping bag. Curious about its contents, I asked Daphne what they had brought. She looked at me sheepishly. "My vitamins," she breathed.

When I peered into the bag, I struggled to hold my composure. I was flabbergasted. In this sack were *twenty-two* bottles of various supplements ranging from melatonin to MSM cream. (MSM [methylsulphonylmethane] is a naturally occurring organic sulphur compound found in all living plant and animal tissues. It is essential for all bodily systems and normal organ functions.) It appeared as if she had been attacked by an overzealous vitamin salesperson. The likelihood that Daphne was benefiting from all these supplements was slim to none. Aside from the potential for side effects resulting from mixing so many different things, the vitamins were of low quality and lacked enzymes to assist in their breakdown. Therefore, it was possible that she was not absorbing them at all, thus essentially wasting her time, effort, and money. I was happy she was open to taking supplements but wanted to assist her in getting the right ones.

I ordered a urine test for Daphne to check her organic acids and assessed her vitamin and mineral levels. She was in need of B-complex and vitamin D. She also needed probiotics and more fatty acids, so we gave her some broad-spectrum probiotics and some flaxseed oil. Because her plan was customized, the client now only needed three supplements instead of twenty-two. This change alone was a huge relief for her.

I had warned Daphne that the vitamins would need two to three weeks to kick in. About one week later, the urgency to move her bowels began to decrease, and she spent less time in a diaper. She also swore off fast food and dairy. Three months went by, and each baby step Daphne made to change her health brought her dramatic improvement. At our sixth session, Daphne informed me she had traveled to visit her daughter the previous week and, surprisingly, had been able to navigate her trip without the use of diapers. This was a huge step.

Daphne decided to stick with her new supplement plan and reaped the benefits, promising that she would not go back to taking bags full of vitamins again.

Are you walking around with a bag of supplements? Are you taking supplements because your neighbor's Aunt Sally's daughter's brother-in-law said they were good for you? If so, contact a professional to help you assess your specific needs. You could really be doing a disservice to your body rather than nurturing it. Also, avoid another common trap—don't heed the advice of vitamin salespeople in chain stores. Most may be well meaning, but they are not nutrition or medical professionals, and this can lead you to purchase vitamins you really don't need. Most importantly, the right supplements can make all the difference for the person suffering from IBD.

Supplements for a Special Digestive System

You may have heard that taking supplements can help control your IBD. But which ones should you take, and how should you take them? More importantly, *why* is it a good idea to look into fortifying your daily diet this way? The average person feels lost among all the choices in a vitamin store. The guide below explains the various options available for the IBD patient and how to take maximum advantage of them.

Why Use Supplements?

People with IBD often suffer from insufficient nutrition due to the illness's digestive constraints. Given the challenges of adequate nutrition intake and absorption, it makes sense for those with IBD to supplement to assist in the metabolism of vital nutrition. Your digestive tract is the gateway for your body's essential nutritional needs, so you definitely want to have a clean, well-nourished colon to prevent disease and malabsorption.

The colon and small intestine are a vital part of the body, because they perform such a significant job. If your colon and small intestine are not functioning properly, as is the case for most with IBD, you are almost guaranteed to experience an overall decline in health. The primary explanation: The colon is the number-one repository for oxidative stress in the body. Oxidative stress on the body changes cells and can damage and change a person's genes. Oxidative stress goes hand in hand with epigenetics, as discussed earlier on page 15. You may hear a great deal in the media about antioxidants and the danger of oxidative stress, but few people know that the majority of oxidative stress and damage is generated in the colon during the final stages of the digestive process.[1]

Therefore, if the bowel is not working to full capacity, you are at a higher risk for developing deficiencies in antioxidant vitamins, such as A, C, and E. A study performed by the American Dietetic Association showed that moderate levels of vitamin C can prevent and treat cancer, a debilitating disease that can be encouraged by free radical damage and excessive oxidative stress.[2]

IBD patients should proactively exercise preventative measures against cancer, because studies have shown that those with Crohn's are eighteen times more likely to be diagnosed with colorectal cancer than the general population. The same study revealed that patients with ulcerative colitis possessed nearly the same risk level.[3] Therefore, it is critical to be mindful of your nutritional intake and to eat foods full of appropriate enzymes, vitamins, and minerals.

From personal and professional experience, I can attest to the benefits of proper use of supplements. In 2009 I conducted a survey of thirty-two of my IBD private practice patients who were using supplements to improve their physiology and decrease symptoms. An average of 92 percent of individual symptoms improved while using probiotics, digestive enzymes, and B vitamins, including fatigue, cramping, vomiting, diarrhea, constipation, and bloating. The use of supplements is imperative for those with IBD, especially given the obvious health challenges these patients face.

 Supplements can be a great addition to your current treatment plan. Double-check all supplements with your physician or pharmacist to avoid negative interactions. You can also find this information on http://www.healthnotes.com. Healthnotes is an independent company that provides information about vitamin, mineral, herb, and drug interactions based on scientific data and studies. Supplements are generally safe to use for most patients with IBD, and the majority of people benefit greatly from combining supplements with diet and lifestyle intervention.

Before You Start: Supplement Survey

When considering a supplement regime, you should ask yourself the following questions:

- What happens to your nutrient intake as you go through different stages of your illness?
- To what level is your digestion is compromised (mild, moderate, or severe)?
- Are you flaring up and unable to eat normally?
- What time would you take your supplements so you do not forget?
- What nutritional deficiencies are your medications causing? (Please refer to the chart on page 27.)

Types of Supplements Commonly Used for IBD

- B vitamins
- charcoal
- digestive enzymes
- garlic
- ginger
- natural pain relievers
- omega-3 fatty acids
- probiotics
- superfoods
- vitamin D
- natural anti-inflammatory herbs or foods, such as bromelain

Recommended Supplement #1: Probiotics

Some people are familiar with probiotics due to their growing popularity in yogurt and numerous claims regarding their improvement of digestion.

Probiotics vs. Antibiotics

Probiotics are the "opposite" of antibiotics and help build up the immune system. Probiotics are composed of "friendly" bacteria, such as *Lactobacillus acidophilus*, *Bifidobacterium*, or *Lactobacillus casei*, which are found in yogurt and fermented yams. They can also be found in soil, known as homeostatic soil organisms (HSO). Probiotics have been used for optimum health for centuries,[4] but in recent decades, the United States has become anti-germ and obsessed with antibiotics, leaving our immune systems more vulnerable to attack and more likely to become antibiotic resistant.

When you are getting sick, your immune system sends out attacker cells, known as antibodies. It is your body's job, with the help of good bacteria, to fight off the unfriendly bacteria that are making you sick. This process allows your immune system to rid the body of infections, naturally. If you see your doctor for a bacterial infection of some sort, you would generally be prescribed an antibiotic. When you are sick with an overabundance of unfriendly bacteria in your gut and then you take an antibiotic, both the bad bacteria *and* the good bacteria your intestines need to maintain health die off.

Taking an antibiotic can leave your digestive tract vulnerable to diseases and illness.

The Benefits of Probiotics

Everyone's bodies contain billions of different bacteria, found in our large and small intestines. Some of the bacteria are good, and some are bad. To maintain optimum health, the recommended ratio is 85 percent friendly bacteria to 15 percent bad bacteria. Sadly, many Americans find that the ratio is actually reversed.[5]

This situation is a breeding ground for an unhealthy body, because without friendly bacteria, the immune system does not function very well at all, and this increases your susceptibility to diseases. Taking probiotics can increase the amount of friendly bacteria in the gut, improving digestive health and promoting overall wellness in the body. Probiotics can be especially helpful for chronic digestive illnesses, such as Crohn's disease, ulcerative colitis, diverticulitis, celiac disease, and irritable bowel syndrome (IBS), as well as other autoimmune disorders like cancer, MS, and lupus.[6]

Probiotics have also been shown to:[7]

- improve digestion
- improve immunity
- lower LDL cholesterol

- reduce risk of cancer
- regulate hormones
- produce vitamins

Why Try Probiotics?

Those with inflammatory bowel disease (IBD) and IBS should take probiotics. In a Polish study of IBS published in the *Lancet*, one hundred people were given lactobacilli, a placebo, or antispasmodic drugs. Astonishingly, nearly 75 percent of those taking lactobacilli reported substantial improvement, compared with only 27 percent taking the drugs and 0 percent taking the placebo.[8] Clearly, a 75 percent success rate with probiotics is far better than a 27 percent rate with pharmaceuticals. Other studies have shown similar results.[9] Probiotics were a key aspect of my own recovery and of the recovery of the majority of my IBD clients. No matter what stage you are in with your disease, you should add them to your treatment regime.

What to Look for When Purchasing a Probiotic

Most commercial probiotics are cultured on dairy, but this is not ideal because many of those afflicted with IBD have dairy allergies or sensitivities. Look for probiotics made from homeostatic soil organisms (HSOs). HSOs are found in soil and are responsible for giving foods the enzymes we need to break them down. See the Resources section for some manufacturers of HSOs.

How to Take Probiotics

Take probiotics on an empty stomach for maximum effect. If you have mild to moderate IBD, start with three probiotics daily for one week. Gradually increase by one capsule per week until you reach six. Remain at six for at least thirty days to adequately repopulate beneficial bacteria, and then decrease by one capsule per week until you are back to three. Remain at three indefinitely as a maintenance dosage.

If you have severe IBD, follow the same protocol above, but increase to nine capsules daily for thirty days and then gradually decrease to a maintenance dosage of four capsules daily.

Recommended Supplement #2: Enzymes

Enzymes are chemical compounds that break down food into smaller particles. These smaller particles, comprised of proteins, turn into amino acids and complex carbohydrates, which turn into simple sugars and convert fat into fatty acids and glycerol. In a healthy system, your liver, pancreas, stomach, and intestines should produce and supply about ten quarts of digestive juices to your digestive tract daily—something that generally doesn't happen for those with IBD.

The body makes three different types of enzymes: indigenous, metabolic, and food. *Metabolic enzymes* allow tissues, cells, and organs to work properly. *Indigenous enzymes* are secreted by the pancreas and small intestine. They also take over when not enough food enzymes are present to complete the job. Finally, *food enzymes* are supplied by what you eat. Abundant enzymes naturally occur in most raw fruits, meats, sprouted nuts, seeds, and vegetables. Many doctors make the mistake of advising the majority of those with IBD to stay away from raw fruits and vegetables, which then decreases enzyme production in the body.

Without enzymes, you cannot break down your food. Your body needs to absorb nutrition just to make enzymes, so a vicious cycle develops for some with IBD. It is a difficult situation. You need nutrition to make enzymes, but if you aren't able to adequately absorb nutrition, you are losing nutrients in addition to limiting further enzyme production. For those with chronic flare-ups, enzyme therapy is essential when you cannot receive sufficient nutrition, especially if you have food sensitivities or allergies or when any inflammation is present in the digestive tract.

Types of Enzyme Supplements You Should Look For

Enzyme-based, anti-inflammatory, whole-food supplements can be an excellent defense against IBD flare-ups because they assist your body in gaining valuable nutrition and allow your body to break down foods more comfortably and naturally. A number of these types of enzyme formulations are available that have shown great benefit for those with IBD. Chapter 7 includes resources for ordering enzymes. Look for a multi-enzyme formula with a combination of all of the following types of enzymes:

- amylase—responsible for converting carbohydrates into simple sugar to use as energy (ATP) to fuel the brain
- bromelain—found in pineapples and papayas, responsible for protein breakdown
- lactase—breaks down naturally occurring sugar found in milk
- lipase—splits fats into three fatty acids and glycerol
- invertase—breaks down sucrose into glucose and fructose

- papain—derived from papaya, digests proteins into peptides and amino acids
- phytase—breaks down phytic acid, the tricky substance in beans that is hard for most people to break down
- protease/peptidase—responsible for the breakdown of amino acids

How to Take Enzymes

Take enzymes each time you eat and as directed by the manufacturer. If you inadvertently consume a food to which you are intolerant or allergic, you may also take enzymes to counteract the reaction. Enzymes are highly recommended for those with IBD, whether the illness is mild, moderate, or severe.

Recommended Supplement #3: Omega-3 Fatty Acids

In the late 1980s Dean Ornish's research on low-fat diets became all the rage. Practically overnight, consumers began demanding foods that were low-fat or fat-free. This concept does have some merit. Saturated fats do not support health and can cause heart disease and contribute to obesity. But some fats are vital, such as omega-3 fatty acids. Ironically, omega-3 fatty acids do the exact opposite job as saturated fats. Foods containing these healthy fatty acids are touted for lowering LDL cholesterol, boosting immunity, and supporting metabolic and cardiovascular functions.

Omega-3 fatty acids have been proven to reduce pain and inflammation in IBD patients as well as those with arthritis.[10] Omega-3s are found in many different foods, including tuna, mackerel, salmon, walnuts, olives, coconut, avocados, sardines, chia, and flaxseed.

Three major types of omega-3 fatty acids are:

1. alpha-linolenic acid (ALA)
2. docosahexaenoic acid (DHA)
3. eicosapentaenoic acid (EPA)

When eaten, ALA is converted into EPA and DHA, the two fatty acids that are primarily used by the body for different processes, such as improving cardiovascular function, lowering blood pressure, and boosting brain function. Moreover, EPA and DHA have anti-inflammatory properties.

How to Take Omega-3 Fatty Acids

Take 1,000 mg of omega-3s daily in the form of flaxseed oil, coconut oil, or fish oil. See Chapter 7 for recommended brands and products. This supplement can be used for mild, moderate, or severe IBD. If fish oil causes or worsens diarrhea, discontinue using it.

Recommended Supplement #4: Garlic

Garlic is an antimicrobial food, meaning it can fight off many forms of infection, whether bacterial, fungal, parasitic, or viral in nature.[11] Allicin is the active constituent in garlic that is responsible for this function.

How to Take Garlic

Consume garlic when you have any type of infection. When the garlic has been removed from the bulb to make a supplement, the allicin content is destroyed; therefore it is best to eat it in its natural state. Eat one to five raw cloves daily for maximum benefit. You can also mince the garlic and infuse it in olive oil to use as salad dressing.

Recommended Supplement #5: Vitamin-B Complex

When I first meet clients, I often hear, "Wow, you have a lot of energy! Where does it come from?" Aside from enthusiasm for my job, my peppiness can be accredited to the high amount of B vitamins I take daily. This is just one of the fantastic benefits of B vitamins, as they also help fight depression and anxiety, assist with bowel movements by increasing muscle contractions in the gut, and even improve your hair, skin, and nails. Each B vitamin plays a different role related to digestion and IBD.

Intrinsic Factor and Vitamin B-12

Ever wonder why having digestive trouble zaps your energy? Vitamin B-12 is necessary for blood formation, high energy levels, growth, and cell division. B-12 is absorbed in the stomach by a process called intrinsic factor. Intrinsic factor works directly with extrinsic factor, which is the absorption of nutrients from food. Without these two processes, the body cannot absorb B-12.

As you age and your body's production of hydrochloric acid slows down, it negatively affects the intrinsic factor, causing you to need more B vitamins. (Hydrochloric acid is produced in the stomach and serves many functions, including assisting in the breakdown of foods as well as providing assistance to the immune system by killing off microbial infections, such as those caused by a bacteria or virus.) Because the typical diet consists of many "enriched foods" that are missing appropriate sources of vitamin B-12, you must assess your B-vitamin intake to ensure optimal digestion.

B vitamins also help assist peristalsis, the musclelike contractions that help waste and nutrition pass through the intestines. A lack of B-vitamin absorption causes this function to slow down, increasing the risk for constipation, especially if the diet lacks fiber and water.

How to Take B Vitamins

Try to find a B-vitamin complex that is whole-food based (refer to Chapter 7 for specific brands), and take as directed. If you need additional energy, you can generally double-up on B vitamins, because they are water soluble and excreted through the urine if consumed in excess amounts.

Recommended Supplement #6: Charcoal

Charcoal is a black powder made from wood or other natural materials by heating them in an airless environment. Charcoal used for health conditions is usually "activated" to make it a very fine powder, which increases its effectiveness. For those with IBD, charcoal can help in the case of an infection or accidental food poisoning. Activated charcoal can chemically attach to, or adsorb, a variety of particles and gases, which makes it ideal for removing potentially toxic substances from the digestive tract. Activated charcoal is not absorbed into the body, so it carries unwanted substances out of the body in the feces. In studies it has been shown to decrease IBD symptoms.[12] It is also thought to help with heartburn and indigestion.

How to Take Charcoal

If you have mild to moderate IBD, take 50 mg daily for two weeks, and then assess how you feel. If you notice a decrease in your symptoms, continue taking 25 mg daily for as long as desired.

Recommended Supplement #7: Multivitamin

For obvious reasons, a multivitamin is recommended. Choose a multivitamin of very high quality to ensure maximum absorption. Look for whole-food-based supplements, which are much better than their synthetic counterparts, because they provide the benefit of enhanced absorption. Increased absorption is key for individuals with IBD, especially someone with food intolerances and nutrient deficiencies. The best supplements should be raw (meaning uncooked) and as close to nature as possible in their makeup. Also, ideal supplements include a built-in probiotic to enhance digestion and boost immunity and digestive enzymes.

How to Take Multivitamins

Take as directed. For maximum absorption, take supplements with food.

Recommended Supplement #8: Vitamin C

Any nutrition professional I have spoken with has always been fond of good old vitamin C, because it protects the immune system so efficiently. Anytime you feel a flare-up coming on, start taking vitamin C to help shorten the length of the infection and the inflammation. A therapeutic dose would be about 3,000 mg daily for an adult and can vary for children depending on their age, weight, and height. Vitamin C also offers many other benefits, such as energy production, improved dental health, and cancer prevention due to its antioxidant properties.

Nature's Painkillers

It is no secret to anyone suffering from IBD that at some point in the course of your illness, you will experience pain. It can quickly go from nonexistent to severe and can vary in frequency and duration. Fortunately, you can naturally alleviate pain in several ways. First and foremost, contact your physician. If your doctor does not deem your situation urgent, you can then utilize the power of nature's medicine cabinet.

Because inflammation in the body causes pain,[13] consider supplementation for IBD to control and to prevent inflammation, and to reduce or diminish discomfort. By approaching this goal with whole-food sources of nutrition, you'll naturally put your body back into a state of health and restore the integrity of your digestive system. Therefore, the following supplements help control pain and lower inflammation at the same time by reducing the overproduction of leukotrienes (a class of small inflammation-promoting molecules produced by cells in response to allergen exposure).

Turmeric

Turmeric is a bright yellow-orange spice touted for its immune system–boosting properties by Native Americans. Therapeutically, it has been proven to treat inflammation in the body. This spice contains the active compound curcumin, which has been proven to be even more effective than anti-inflammatory drugs, without the undesirable side effects.[14]

How to take: Take 500 mg, one to three times daily, as needed for pain. It is recommended for those with mild, moderate, or severe IBD.

Boswellia

Also known as Indian Frankincense, boswellia is noted for its anti-inflammatory properties. Although most studies of its effects pertained to subjects with arthritis, they indicated that boswellia helps improve blood flow and circulation to inflamed tissue, thus decreasing pain. Even though this research was not specific to IBD, many practitioners presume this herb is also good for the intestines based on the current information available.

How to use: Purchase boswellia as a cream containing 200 to 400 mg, which can be rubbed directly over the lower abdomen for maximum absorption in the intestines. Apply as needed for pain up to three times daily. This cream is also effective for those who have rheumatoid arthritis. It can be used for mild, moderate, or severe IBD, although it is most effective for mild to moderate patients.

IsoOxygene

An extract found in hops called IsoOxygene has been found to work well as a painkiller, without the nasty side effects that often come from prescription drugs. COX-2, an enzyme responsible for inflammation and pain can be inhibited by the use of Isooxygene, one of the most potent natural COX-2 inhibitors. In Patrick Holford's *Optimum Nutrition Bible* he cites a study in which two tablets of ibuprofen inhibited COX-2 by 62 percent, whereas IsoOxygene achieved a 56 percent rate of inhibition.

Not only is it almost as effective as ibuprofen, but it also doesn't have the negative gut-related side effects of anti-inflammatory drugs. This is because ibuprofen also inhibits the COX-1 enzyme (often called the "good" COX because it produces prostacyclin, a substance that protects the lining of the gut), whereas the hop extract does not.

How to take: Take 1,500 mg as needed.

Ginger

Because it contains a plethora of antioxidants, ginger really packs a therapeutic punch. This potent root is widely recognized for its anti-nausea and anti-inflammatory properties, along with its ability to control pain.[15]

How to take: Ginger can be taken orally (500 to 2,000 mg daily) for inflammation reduction as a capsule or made into a tea to control nausea. For tea, add a two-inch strip of ginger to four cups of water. Bring to a boil. Remove from heat and allow to steep for about ten to fifteen minutes. Remove the ginger strip and serve warm.

Chapter 6

· · · · · · · · · · · · · ·

Essential IBD Resources

This chapter is your one-stop shop for all your digestive wellness needs. It includes:

- information on foods that might be well suited to your diet based on your blood type
- a Menu Planner
- a sample allergen-free menu
- contact information for helpful diagnostic laboratories
- listings for helpful health websites

The activities are designed to allow you to utilize the information that you have learned thus far and put it all together. To ensure maximum benefit from reading this book, first consult with the information listed for your blood type (see "Eating for Your Blood Type" on the next page) to evaluate the foods that are likely best for your metabolism as well as foods you should avoid, and then use the Menu Planner to design your ideal diet based upon what you have already learned from reading this book.

Tiffany's Story

Tiffany was a busy mom who strived to take excellent care of her children, home, career—everyone and everything except for herself! She had been diagnosed with Crohn's disease two years before I met her. After suffering for more than a year, and after much trial and error, she had intuitively decided that she should avoid dairy. After removing milk, cheese, butter, and yogurt from her diet, she showed marked improvement in her digestive symptoms, such as diarrhea and nausea. As long as she kept dairy out of her diet, most of the time she seemed to feel just fine.

Although omitting dairy had made somewhat of a difference for her, Tiffany still had symptoms on occasion and could not figure out why. She had come to consult with me to determine why her symptoms were still lingering. Initially suspecting she had another food intolerance, cross-sensitivity, or an entirely different issue, I asked Tiffany to log a food diary for a week. After looking over her food diary, I wasn't surprised at her persisting symptoms. I noted that she ate out for most meals, and when she did, she was consuming dairy, either purposely or inadvertently. She almost never cooked at home, and when she did, it was frozen, convenience food which was problematic, as several of them had dairy hidden inside.

After I worked with Tiffany on menu planning, it became easier for her to see that she could not only save herself a lot of time and effort but also a lot of money. Most important, after two weeks of consuming home-cooked meals, her digestive issues subsided even further. I suspected the dairy that she was accidentally eating had been the culprit. On her third week of eating from home, she reported that nausea had not plagued her in nearly two weeks, and, for the first time in almost a year, she had normal stools.

For Tiffany, recovery was all about slowing down, cooking more, paying attention to her food, discovering hidden sources of dairy, and getting back to basics. Once she was able to embrace this approach, her digestion improved greatly—and remained that way.

Eating for Your Blood Type

The blood-type diet was established by Dr. Peter D'Adamo. As of this writing, I am unable to locate any medical journal studies demonstrating the benefit of this diet; however many other significant case studies have indicated its effectiveness. In a case study by Dr. D'Adamo, out of 3,310 blood-type diet participants, more than 1,200 subjects reported positive changes in digestion, metabolism, and energy. They also indicated that they experienced significant increases in energy and success with stabilizing their metabolism.[1]

Eating for your blood type is based on the following premise: Each blood type originated during a different time period, so you can assume that the foods that you would best assimilate would be the staples of that era.

Here is an example: Blood type A originated between 25,000 and 15,000 BC. During this time, people were beginning to practice organized agriculture and began eating a diet that contained less animal fat and more fruits, vegetables, and grains. This differs from the diet recommended for someone with type O blood, who does better with meats, because this blood type originated when people were still primarily hunters and gatherers.

Keep in mind that every person is an individual. No two diets will be completely alike, of course. Experiment with this diet to determine its effectiveness for you. I have worked with many clients in my practice who have found it helpful. The following tables will guide you in choosing foods that may be most appropriate for you based on your blood type. They also describe personality traits often common to people of each blood type—whether you are type O, A, B, or AB—as well as some aspects of health that might be problematic for each type.

▍Type O Information (Years of Origin: 30,000–25,000 BC)

(Chart is adapted from the Institute for Integrative Nutrition Blood Type Work Sheet.)

MANNERISMS	FOODS TO CONSUME	UNSUPPORTIVE FOODS TO METABOLISM	HEALTH RISK	HEALTH WEAKNESS
Strong	Meat	Wheat	Inflammation	Low tolerance to new environments/diets
Hunter	Protein	Corn	Arthritis	Overactive immune system
Leader	Fruits	Baked goods	Blood clotting disorders	Underactive immune system

(cont'd.)

▌Type O Information (Years of origin: 30,000–25,000 BC) (cont'd.)

MANNERISMS	FOODS TO CONSUME	UNSUPPORTIVE FOODS TO METABOLISM	HEALTH RISK	HEALTH WEAKNESS
Self-reliant	Vegetables	Lentils	Overacidity	
Goal-oriented		Navy beans	Ulcers	
		Kidney beans		

▌Type A Information (Years of Origin 25,000–15,000 BC)

MANNERISMS	FOODS TO CONSUME	UNSUPPORTIVE FOODS TO METABOLISM	HEALTH RISK	HEALTH WEAKNESS
Adapts well to changes in environment	Vegetables	Meat	Anemia	Sensitive digestive tract
Little need for animal food	Tofu	Dairy	Cancer	Immune system vulnerability
Metabolism of nutrients is optimal	Grains	Kidney beans	Liver and gallbladder disorders	Prone to microbial invasion
	Beans	Lima beans	Type 1 diabetes	
	Fish	Wheat	Heart disease	

▌Type B Information (Years of Origin 10,000–15,000 BC)

MANNERISMS	FOODS TO CONSUME	UNSUPPORTIVE FOODS TO METABOLISM	HEALTH RISK	HEALTH WEAKNESS
Nomad	Meat	Chicken	Fatigue	None
Flexible	Dairy	Corn	Diabetes	
Creative	Grains	Lentils	Auto-immune disorders	
	Fruits	Peanuts	MS	
	Vegetables	Sesame	Lupus	

▌Type AB Information (Year of Origin: 2500 BC)

MANNERISMS	FOODS TO CONSUME	UNSUPPORTIVE FOODS TO METABOLISM	HEALTH RISK	HEALTH WEAKNESS
Rare	Meat	Corn	Cancer	Sensitive digestive tract
Enigmatic	Seafood	Buckwheat	Anemia	Hyposensitive immune system responses generating microbial invasions
Mysterious	Tofu	Seeds	Heart disease	
Highly sensitive	Fruits			
	Vegetables			

Enter your relevant blood-type information at the top of the Menu Planner on the next page where it asks for your "Blood Type," "Good Foods Based on Blood Type," and "Foods to Avoid Based on Blood Type." Use this first section of the Menu Planner as a reference when trying to determine which foods to choose when shopping and preparing meals. See how you feel while on the blood-type diet, and indicate any symptoms in the Menu Planner.

Your Menu Planner

To design your ideal diet, compile all the data you generated from your blood type and any food-intolerance testing or elimination-diet results. Look through the recipes featured in Chapter 7 of this book to find which work best for you.

Use this chart to plan out your meals. The first step to stress-free cooking is planning. Planning helps you dissolve your digestive troubles by preventing you from eating foods that are unsupportive to your health goals. Try it out! Plan out your meals for a week, and note whether you have a change in symptoms. You should see positive results if you are sticking to an appropriate dietary regime. Jot down any digestive problems, and look for a pattern. Sometimes you may be eating a food that is affecting you, and this chart is also a means to pinpoint the issues that food intolerances can cause.

Your Menu Planner

BLOOD TYPE: _____

FOOD ALLERGIES/ INTOLERANCES	GOOD FOODS BASED ON BLOOD TYPE	FOODS TO AVOID BASED ON BLOOD TYPE

	MONDAY	TUESDAY	WEDNESDAY	THURSDAY	FRIDAY	SATURDAY	SUNDAY
Breakfast							
Any digestive symptoms? Y or N							
Lunch							
Any digestive symptoms? Y or N							

(cont'd.)

	MONDAY	TUESDAY	WEDNESDAY	THURSDAY	FRIDAY	SATURDAY	SUNDAY
Dinner							
Any digestive symptoms? Y or N							

Sample Allergen-Free Menu

This menu is free of four potential allergens—gluten, dairy, soy, and eggs. It is suitable for pescetarians.

	MONDAY	TUESDAY	WEDNESDAY	THURSDAY
Breakfast	• Nature's Path Organic Crunchy Vanilla Sunrise Cereal with vanilla almond milk, organic blueberries, pecans	• Tropical smoothie with coconut milk, mango juice, banana, pineapple, and lemon juice • Serve with Ener-G Light Brown Rice bread and organic apricot jam	• Sweet potato pancakes topped with natural maple syrup and strawberries • (Pancake batter: 1 sweet potato, grated, 1 mashed banana, 2 tablespoons cornstarch, 2 tablespoons onion powder, salt, pepper)	• Apple cinnamon millet porridge or oatmeal • (1 cup cooked millet or oatmeal, 1 whole apple, grated; ½ cup toasted walnuts, 1 teaspoon vanilla, 2 tablespoons maple syrup, 1 teaspoon cinnamon, pinch nutmeg, pinch allspice)

(cont'd.)

	MONDAY	TUESDAY	WEDNESDAY	THURSDAY
Lunch	• Cod crunchy tacos made with organic corn or brown-rice taco shells filled with avocado, romaine, scallions, tomatoes, and sautéed onions and peppers	• Pineapple pizzas • (Enjoy Life bagels topped with tomato sauce and pineapple slices) • Red pepper slices with vinaigrette dressing • So Delicious coconut blueberry yogurt	• Bean salad with red pepper, vinaigrette, and onion over wild rice • Dried fruit and toasted walnut and coconut trail mix with organic dark chocolate chips	• Almond butter and grape jelly sandwich on Enjoy Life Bread • Natural potato chips • Guacamole over simple salad (romaine, scallions)
Dinner	• Bean taquitos (baked corn tortillas with refried beans rolled into cigars) • Top with salsa verde • Naked baked potato	• Grilled tuna steaks over steamed spaghetti squash • Grilled asparagus • Sweet potato fries	• Fish and veggie shish kebab with peppers, onions, and halibut • Fruity shishkebab with peaches and plums • Fried brown rice	• Grilled mackerel with pineapple salsa over brown rice • Roasted broccoli and cauliflower with olive oil, sea salt, and pepper

Mindful Eating

Mindful eating is the practice of being aware of your food choices and how you eat your meals. When you are not conscious of your diet, think about how this can affect you. Depending on your level of awareness around food, you may tend to choose foods that wouldn't bother you one day but might the next. For example, let's say you have a routine that lacks proper planning. You are at the office, and you are going from one meeting to the next. Because you weren't thinking of lunch, by the time the meeting has come to a close, you are starving. You can no longer wait to eat, because your blood-sugar levels are plummeting, so you decide to reach for the closest thing. Unfortunately, it is none other than your arch-nemesis: the candy bar. Eating in this manner is not considered mindful, because you did not take the time to anticipate this situation.

My colleague Dr. Robert Lichtenstein says that mindful eating encompasses not only planning your meals but also what you are doing *while* you are actually *eating* your meals. For instance, it is not a great idea to watch TV, to read a newspaper, or to do anything other than concentrating on your food during mealtimes.

When you are distracting yourself from the task at hand—digestion—you are sending a signal to the brain telling it to switch off the digestive process. Therefore, you will not digest your food properly, resulting in malabsorption of nutrients. When you are not paying attention to your food intake, you are also more likely to overeat. Don't think so? Here is an example: A study was conducted in which movie-theater patrons were offered free popcorn. All the participants were very happy to be offered the treat and greedily ate the large buttery-flavored tubs of kernels while watching the movie. Not one moviegoer complained, and some even asked for seconds.

After the flick, the patrons were then offered another tub. "This popcorn is fresh," one participant commented. Another tasted the new popcorn and noticed that the original serving had been stale. One by one, the movie-goers realized they had *all* eaten entire tubs of three-day-old popcorn. In the trance of movie watching they had not been paying any attention to consuming their snack, and not *one* of the participants realized their snack was stale. Amazingly, we really don't always realize how much of an impact ignoring our food intake can have. You can really see the importance of mindful eating.

Mindful Eating and IBD

People with IBD must be mindful of their eating at least 90 percent of the time. Keep in mind that no one is perfect, so be gentle with yourself, especially in the beginning. You may feel that this large percentage is difficult to achieve, but to live symptom free and reduce stress in your life, you should be aware of what nutritionists call the 90/10 rule: Ninety percent of the time eat what is good, and then 10 percent of the time you can eat something that is not so great without terrible consequences, such as a flare-up. This ratio does vary by individual. For instance, someone with severe casein intolerance may not be able to properly tolerate even the smallest amount of dairy, so avoidance of this protein should be practiced religiously to prevent potentially dangerous health-threatening consequences.

The rewards for practicing mindful eating are far greater than the slight inconveniences. For one thing, you'll begin to prefer healthier foods, a phenomenon known as the crowding-out theory. If you simply begin adding more healthy foods into your diet, by process of natural selection, less-healthy foods are then taken out of the diet. Secondly, as you change your eating habits, you begin to notice how eating differently is affecting not only your physical stamina but also your emotional well-being. Today's world is very fast paced. One thing you may forget to do is to stop and actually chew your foods properly. Typically people who eat quickly are always rushing and hurrying to get to their next event. I see this commonly with those whom I counsel in private practice.

Mindful-Eating Exercise

Spend two weeks completing a study that will allow you to determine how your digestion affects you, especially when you're being mindful of your food intake.

For week one of the experiment, prepare all or most of your meals from home. Make a plan to eat all your meals without any distractions—no TV, no computer, no reading. Instead, try to have a relaxing dinner with friends or family. Take the time to reflect how you feel physically before and after your meals. Keep a food diary throughout this process to gain more accurate insight as to how eating in this manner affects you.

For week two of the experiment, feel free to eat on the run and in front of the TV. Outside of keeping a diary to record your symptoms, don't pay much attention to your food intake. See how the two weeks compare to one another. What changes did you notice?

How Much Should You Chew?

Often in our busy, fast-paced lives, we tend to forget that we should slow down and enjoy life. Interestingly, the importance of chewing is one of the elements I have found that has escaped people's minds surrounding digestion. Many people today eat as if they are competing in some sort of food race to the finish line. This approach is not a sound one because digestion begins at the mouth and ends at the anus. If your teeth don't properly grind up your food, you will have problems with your intestinal tract, such as inflammation. Thirty chews per mouthful of food are recommended. When you begin eating, your body produces amylase (a digestive enzyme) in your saliva to assist in breaking down your food properly so your body can assimilate energy directly into your cells. If you do not take the time to chew adequately, you will miss out on the production of those enzymes. This can significantly affect your ability to digest food and may even result in a flare-up because the job of digestion is left to your stomach and then finally to your intestines. Leaving digestion to these organs is not ideal because much of your nutrient absorption occurs along the walls of your intestines, and food that is not yet broken down cannot be absorbed properly.

It has been reported that eating while stressed or on the run can cause food intolerance. If you do not spend adequate time chewing, you will notice a decline in your overall digestion speed and energy levels. As your digestion speed slows down, your ability to break down certain foods is inhibited, and this can lead to the development of a food intolerance.

The Chewing Challenge

For one meal, record how many times you chew each bite. Try putting your fork back down on the plate to force yourself slow down a bit. You can also try using children's chopsticks (these typically resemble a small, one-piece set of tongs) which are easier to use than those for adults. However, they deliver smaller bites, which slows down the eating process enough to allow you to chew more than you would if you were to use traditional flatware. If you have IBD, slowing down is very important because it allows your sensitive digestive tract the time it needs to successfully digest your food.

Have some fun with the chewing challenge! Look for children's chopsticks online; they come in cute designs.

To Sum It Up

We have now reached the beginning of the recipe section. At this point, my hope is that you have learned as much as possible about IBD and helping yourself. I hope you implement the exercises in *The IBD Healing Plan and Recipe Book* and start discovering your own unique path to wellness. Carpe diem! You have one life to live, and it is waiting for you. Motivation comes from doing, so the more you do to get well, the more motivated you will be to remain well and to take the best care of yourself. And why not give yourself extra TLC—you deserve it!

If approaching your IBD alone seems too daunting, please ask for help. Many qualified naturopaths and nutritionists can assist you with implementing the suggestions in this book. Have your trusted practitioner read through this book so that they can become familiar with the treatment protocols and how to implement them with you. Just take one step at a time, and before you know it, you'll be off and running toward a healthy life.

Here are my final words of wisdom. I hope you will find a little humor in some of these, as I think they are vital for sticking to the IBD Healing Plan.

Christie's IBD Words of Wisdom

1. **Embrace your wellness journey,** and try to discover what IBD is trying to teach you. My IBD taught me to make lemonade when life handed me what I thought were lemons. Enjoy learning about your body along the way, and treat it well, because it is the only one you've got.

2. **Laugh at yourself.** Let's face it, IBD can be painful, but it can also be downright embarrassing. You know what I am talking about. Trying to cover up flatulence during a work meeting does not always make for a delightful experience. If only people knew what IBD people go through. But you must laugh to

keep your sanity in the end. After all, the little kid in you may think it was funny that you farted at dinner.

3. **Don't let your disease stop you.** At times you will be more comfortable at home, and by all means, honor that. But you can do anything you want, even if you have IBD. Don't be afraid to go out and live life. There will always be a bathroom, a menu you can eat, and so on. Remember to do a little prep work in advance to make your life easier. This habit will make you more organized in the long run—an added bonus.

4. **Don't allow yourself to catch a case of the "Screw its."** This advice is my personal favorite. Pardon my French, but clients always laugh at this one, and the theory behind this is very true. When you are down and out, sometimes you just throw your hands up and say "Screw it," right? When I see clients do that, usually they cease to take care of themselves, because frustration prevents them from caring. Have you ever felt this way when at your wit's end with your IBD? A lot of us have. It is important to acknowledge this fact: Yes, IBD can really stink sometimes (ummm, perhaps literally), and it is okay to get angry. Expressing your emotions is healthy. But please limit all pity parties to a short time frame. Life is too short to be negative. In the long term, the stress won't help your IBD, so focus on being thankful for what you do have. No matter how small the list may be at first, with a little practice, you can really change your mindframe to be more positive.

5. **Do silly things to smile.** My dad and I joked around often when I was sick. I even went as far as making up a catchy but ridiculously stupid song about spending my life in a bath-room. When my disease made me angry, I would sing the silly song, and then I couldn't help but crack up. My co-workers knew the lyrics, and when I had a bad day, they would sing right along with me. One word for that experience: hysterical.

I hope you got a chuckle from the list of things I have learned over the years. I truly hope my five final tips of IBD wisdom are helpful for you.

Reading this book should give you fresh insight on how to take care of your IBD. I hope it allows you to eradicate any food sensitivities that have contributed to your disorder, as well as to find ways to cope with the situation at large. Knowledge is power, so the more you learn about coping with IBD, the more successful you will be in regaining and basking in optimum health. From the bottom of my heart, I wish you luck with your disease. Keep learning, keep loving, keep healing.

To your health!

Chapter 7

. . . .

The Recipe Corner

The recipes in this section are designed with your delicate digestive system in mind. Almost all are free of the eight most common allergens. This is particularly helpful if you discover that you do possess certain food intolerances; you will still be able to make amazing and healthy meals by following these recipes. If you are having a flare-up, please see the section within this chapter called "Safe Foods for a Flare-Up" for some specific recommendations. Happy cooking!

> **Test Your Own Recipes**
> You can find out if your own recipes are anti-inflammatory by entering them into the free website http://www.nutritiondata.com. The site is a lot of fun! It will even print out a "Nutrition Facts" label for your recipe, just like the ones on the back of packaged products.

Erick's Story

Erick was diagnosed with ulcerative colitis at the age of twenty-four and had survived on a typical bachelor's diet of beer, chips, Gatorade, and hot wings. It became apparent that this diet was not working out after his doctor advised him to drop twenty pounds, stop drinking, and to see a therapist. Erick had just gotten out of the hospital when we had our first visit; fortunately, he had made it through a bad flare-up with his intestines intact.

Erick had contacted me to learn how to cook for his compromised digestion. We needed to start with the basics, going over things like kitchen setup and which utensils and equipment were needed. He even helped me test some of the recipes for this book.

I taught Erick to make smoothies, soups, steamed vegetables, and congee. Congee is excellent for a flare-up, since it does not require very much effort to break it down. It can be made from any grain by cooking it in a slow cooker overnight. Meat can be easily transformed by adding some spices, such as cumin and curry, and roasting or grilling it. The more tricks he learned, the faster and more efficient Erick became in the kitchen.

Erick discovered so much joy in cooking that he decided to enroll in culinary school. His motivation was refreshing. He stopped seeing his therapist, lost thirty pounds, and is truly in love with his life now. Cooking not only his tummy, but his soul as well.

A Note Regarding the Nutritional Information in the Recipes

The nutritional data for the recipes in this book are calculated based on the DV, or Daily Value, established by the National Academy of Sciences in 1998; accordingly, if a recipe has 100 percent of the Daily Value of vitamin C, for example, it contains 60 mg of vitamin C per serving.

Sea salt is recommended vs. iodized table salt as it contains the minerals that we with IBD—especially when flaring or dehydrated— lose at a more rapid rate, like potassium, magnesium, sodium, and chloride. Not to mention that iodized salt is highly refined and digests poorly. Look for pink- or blue-toned Celtic sea salts, as they are "real" sea salt. Don't be tricked into buying "sea salt" that is white, as white sea salt has been stripped of almost all of its minerals, making it refined and of poor quality.

A Note Regarding Organic Foods

I recommend using organic whenever possible, and please use extra care when choosing organic eggs, strawberries, peaches, apples, and spinach. Check out the "Dirty Dozen" and the "Clean Fifteen" list on the Environmental Working Group's website (http://www.ewg.org

/foodnews/guide) to learn which produce must absolutely be organic to avoid increased exposure to pesticides. There are some circumstances where it is okay to buy nonorganic produce as per the "Clean Fifteen" list, but for optimum nutrition always choose organic.

It is very important to always choose organic greens, as leafy vegetables are the most heavily pesticide-ridden crops. The eggs will always be more nutritious when organic, making this an important choice.

A Note Regarding Healthy Fish, Meat, and Poultry

Choose meat that is organic and grass fed. Grass-fed meat is much more nutritious and contains important anti-inflammatory omega-3s. Omega-3s are needed in abundance for those with IBD, so seek out beef, chicken, and turkey, all of which are high in these healthy fats. Organic, grass-fed meats can be found in most health-food stores and through some community-supported farms. For a list of community farms in your area, check http://www.eatwellguide.org. If you cannot find grass-fed meat in your area, some traditional grocers do carry meat that is at least free of antibiotics and hormones. It is not grass fed, but it is still a good option.

All fish and seafood should be wild caught and *never* farm raised. Farm-raised fish are often diseased due to the unnatural methods in which the fish are raised. Farm-raised fish almost always contain dyes to make the fish look healthy. If fish needs food coloring to make it look "normal," this is something to heed warning to. Beware of tilapia, which has taken on some popularity in the recent years, as it is *always* farm raised and should not be included in your diet for this reason. Wild-caught fish and seafood, especially salmon and shrimp, are high in the popular, newly found antioxidant, astaxanthin, and this substance is what gives them their healthy, pink hue. Its health benefits are still widely unknown, but what has been discovered thus far is incredible. For example, it contains lots of oxygen-promoting qualities that make it highly effective for disease prevention.

Breakfast may be considered the most important meal of the day, but for many people with digestive problems, it is the least desirable time to eat. If you are not hungry in the morning, evaluate your eating habits. Oftentimes, people don't have a morning appetite because they eat dinner too late in the evening—say, after 6:00 PM—or they snack before bedtime.

You should aim to have no food after 6:30 PM. This gives your stomach ample time to begin digestion *before* bedtime, which will also help you get restful sleep. When you eat late, your body is digesting food while you slumber. This isn't good because nighttime is the time to give all your systems a rest.

People with IBD frequently experience flare-ups in the mornings, so eating a gentle-on-the-stomach breakfast will help restore energy levels. These recipes are both soothing to the stomach and pleasing to the taste buds.

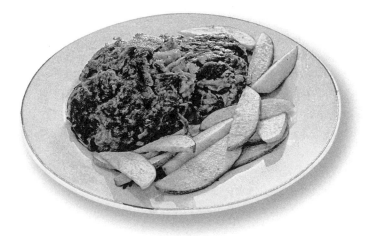

Sweet Potato Pancakes

Love sweet potatoes with dinner? How about breakfast? They are high in vitamin A, which benefits your immune system, skin, and eyesight. Serve these breakfast cakes with maple syrup or unsweetened applesauce, just as you would regular pancakes. There is egg in this recipe, but you can replace it with a substitute, half of a mashed banana, or ½ cup apple sauce.

1 large sweet potato, peeled and finely grated
1 egg
2 tablespoons brown rice flour
1 tablespoon garlic powder
1 tablespoon onion powder
Salt and pepper to taste
1–2 teaspoons coconut or olive oil

Place all the ingredients except the oil in a medium bowl and combine well with your hands until thoroughly blended. Take a small handful of batter (about ¼ cup) and form into pancakes, about ¼-inch thick. You should have about 8 small pancakes.

Melt the oil in a medium-sized nonstick skillet over medium heat. Place the pancakes in the pan in a single layer, making sure to leave a bit of space between each one. Cover the skillet and reduce the heat to medium low. Cook until browned, about 5 minutes. Flip and cook another 5 minutes. You may have to make in 2 batches, as not all of the pancakes will fit in the skillet at once. Serve immediately.

Free of
casein, corn, dairy, eggs, fish, gluten, nuts, soy

Prep time
10 minutes

Total time
20 minutes

Makes
4 servings

Per Serving
Calories: 113
Calories from fat: 33
Total fat: 4 g
Saturated fat: 3 g
Cholesterol: 0 mg
Sodium: 22 mg
Carbohydrates: 19 g
Fiber: 3 g
Sugars: 2 g
Protein: 2 g
Vitamin A: 95% DV
Vitamin C: 2% DV
Calcium: 4% DV
Iron: 3% DV

Carob Chip Banana Pancakes

These are a decadent treat and taste similar to chocolate-chip pancakes. If you have never tried carob before, this recipe will allow you to experiment with it. Carob may be a bit too rich if you are flaring up, so save this yummy recipe for a time when you are feeling great.

1 cup of gluten-free carob chip or allergen-free chocolate chip pancake mix (I recommend Cherrybrook Farms brand)
½ cup vanilla rice milk or coconut milk
¼ cup mashed ripe banana
1 teaspoon flaxseed
1–2 teaspoons coconut oil
Maple syrup to taste (optional)
Fresh berries (optional)
Crushed almonds or pecans (optional)

Free of
casein, dairy, eggs, fish, gluten, nuts, soy

Prep time
5 minutes

Total time
11 minutes

Makes
3 large or 6 small pancakes

Place the pancake mix, milk, banana, and flaxseed oil in a serving bowl and mix gently, until just incorporated. Do not overmix.

Heat the oil in a large nonstick skillet over medium-high heat. Add ¼ cup of the batter per pancake to the skillet, leaving enough room for them to expand. Cook in batches if necessary. Cook for 3 minutes. Flip and cook another 3 minutes or until golden brown.

Serve with maple syrup, berries, and/or nuts.

Per 6-inch Pancake (Without Syrup or Toppings)
Calories: 324
Calories from fat: 81
Total fat: 9 g
Saturated fat: 3 g
Cholesterol: 0 mg
Sodium: 3 mg
Carbohydrates: 252 g
Fiber: 29 g
Sugar: 5 g
Protein: 1 g
Vitamin A: 1% DV
Vitamin C: 3% DV
Calcium: 57% DV
Iron: 2% DV

"Coco-nutty" Almond Pancakes

Finely chopped almonds serve as a flour for these delicious, slightly sweet coco-nutty pancakes. I love to eat these with bananas and raspberries on top and with a drizzle of real maple syrup.

½ cup finely chopped almonds
1¾ cups gluten-free baking flour
1 whole, ripe banana, mashed
¼ cup carob powder (optional)
1 tablespoon nonaluminum baking powder
½ teaspoon salt
1½ cups almond, rice, or soy milk
¼ cup coconut oil
1–2 teaspoons coconut oil
Maple syrup or honey (optional)

Mix all the dry ingredients together in a bowl. In a separate bowl, add the wet ingredients. Pour the wet ingredients into the dry ingredients and stir well.

Heat the vegetable oil in a large nonstick skillet or griddle. Pour ¼ cup of batter per pancake into the skillet, leaving enough space between them to spread. Cook in batches if necessary. Cook for 4 minutes. Flip and cook another 2 minutes, until lightly browned. Serve warm, top with maple syrup or honey.

Free of
casein, corn, dairy, eggs, gluten, soy

Prep time
10 minutes

Total time
10 minutes

Makes
4 servings

Per Serving (Without Topping)
Calories: 448
Calories from fat: 144
Total fat: 16 g
Saturated fat: 3 g
Cholesterol: 0 mg
Sodium: 44 mg
Carbohydrates: 67 g
Fiber: 6 g
Sugars: 5 g
Protein: 12 g
Vitamin A: 4% DV
Vitamin C: 4% DV
Calcium: 22% DV
Iron: 15% DV

Sweet Potato Strudel

Protein-packed quinoa flakes and almonds act as your topping in this tasty new spin on breakfast. This dish is pretty versatile—I like to make it at all times of the day. Sweet potatoes are easy to digest, making them a wonderful food for those with IBD.

2 sweet potatoes
½ cup orange juice
¼ cup maple syrup
¼ cup chopped dried apricots
½ cup toasted quinoa flakes or oats if tolerated
½ cup toasted almonds (optional)

Preheat oven to 350°F.

Place sweet potatoes on baking tray. Poke holes using a fork all over potatoes to allow air to escape and put on a baking sheet. Bake for 1 hour.

About 10 minutes before potatoes are done, heat a small saucepan over medium-low heat. Add the orange juice and maple syrup and stir to combine. Add the dried apricot and cook for about 5 minutes, stirring frequently. If using, add the toasted quinoa flakes and almonds to mixture.

To serve, cut sweet potatoes in half and pour the maple mixture over the top.

Free of
casein, corn, dairy, eggs, fish, gluten, soy

Prep time
10 minutes

Total time
1 hour, 10 minutes

Makes
2 servings

Per Serving
Calories: 375
Calories from fat: 90
Total fat: 11 g
Saturated fat: 1 g
Cholesterol: 0 mg
Sodium: 81 mg
Carbohydrates: 63 g
Fiber: 8 g
Sugars: 24 g
Protein: 10 g
Vitamin A: 383% DV
Vitamin C: 31% DV
Calcium: 11% DV
Iron: 16% DV

Allie's Applesauce Bread

Applesauce bread was a favorite breakfast treat for my client Allie, and she did not want to give it up. I did a little modifying to eliminate the gluten and sugar, and Allie loved the outcome. I bet you will, too.

¼ cup unsweetened applesauce
2 teaspoons baking powder
1 teaspoon baking soda
¼ teaspoon salt
1½ cups filtered water
½ teaspoon xylitol or raw sugar
2 cups gluten-free baking mix

Preheat oven to 350°F.

Combine the flour, baking powder, baking soda, and salt in a large bowl. In another bowl, combine the applesauce, water, and xylitol and mix until just blended. Add wet ingredients to the dry, and stir to combine. Be careful not to over-mix.

Pour the batter into an 8 x 4–inch loaf pan lined with parchment paper. Bake for 30 minutes or until knife comes out clean. Bread should be golden brown when fully baked. Cool before removing from the pan.

Free of
casein, corn, fish, gluten, milk, nuts and soy

Prep time
10 minutes

Total time
42 minutes

Makes
1 loaf (12 slices)

Per Slice
Calories: 99
Calories from fat: 6
Total fat: less than 1 g
Saturated fat: 0 g
Cholesterol: 0 mg
Sodium: 6 mg
Carbohydrates: 19 g
Fiber: 1.25 g
Sugars: 0 g
Protein: 2 g
Vitamin A: 12% DV
Vitamin C: 32% DV
Calcium: 5% DV
Iron: 2% DV

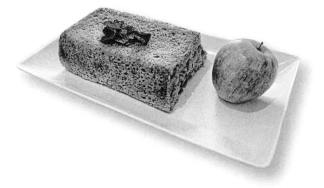

Poached Eggs with Honey Mustard Spinach

I am really big on getting my clients to eat greens, starting with breakfast. Dark, leafy greens such as spinach are an excellent source of vitamins A, C, and E and contain a wide variety of phyto-chemicals, as well as minerals. This dish is very anti-inflammatory.

4 large eggs

1 small red onion, diced

½ red bell pepper, diced

10 ounces fresh baby spinach, chopped

2 tablespoons olive oil

1 tablespoon red wine vinegar

2 teaspoons Dijon mustard

1 teaspoon paprika

Salt and pepper to taste

Free of
casein, corn, dairy, fish, gluten, nuts, soy

Prep time
5 minutes

Total time
15 minutes

Makes
4 servings

Per Serving
Calories: 152
Calories from fat: 79
Total fat: 9 g
Saturated fat: 2 g
Cholesterol: 141 mg
Sodium: 225 mg
Carbohydrates: 11 g
Fiber: 6 g
Sugars: 3 g
Protein: 11 g
Vitamin A: 383% DV
Vitamin C: 52% DV
Calcium: 23% DV
Iron: 22% DV

Fill a large saucepan three quarters full. Heat over high heat until it comes to a boil. Gently crack eggs into water and poach for 4–5 minutes.

While waiting for the water to boil, heat the oil in a medium skillet. Add the onions and peppers and cook for 2–3 minutes, until soft. Add the spinach, gently stirring until barely wilted, about 1 minute. Set aside.

In a small bowl, whisk together the oil, vinegar, mustard, and paprika. Add salt and pepper. Stir the dressing into the spinach.

Divide the spinach mixture on four plates and top with a poached egg.

Granola and Yogurt Parfait

This excellent granola is packed with healthy grains that will give you long-lasting energy. The star grain is quinoa, which is high in amino acids, the building block of protein. Quinoa is one of the few grains considered to be a complete protein. I like to eat it with soy or blueberry coconut yogurt.

¼ cup of honey

2 teaspoons vanilla extract or the seeds from
    2 vanilla beans

2½ cups quinoa flakes

½ cup golden raisins

2 tablespoons chopped dried figs

3 teaspoons pumpkin seeds (pepitas)

2 cups of brown rice cereal

½ cup apple, grated

Preheat oven to 350°F.

Heat the honey in a medium sauce pan over low heat. Once heated through, roll in the quinoa flakes, and stir gently until well coated. Spread the quinoa on a lightly oiled baking sheet and bake until golden brown, about 15 minutes. Remove from oven and allow to cool.

Meanwhile, put the remaining ingredients in a mixing bowl. Stir in the cooled quinoa flakes. Store in an airtight container in the pantry.

Free of
casein, corn, dairy, eggs, gluten, nuts, soy

Prep time
5 minutes

Total time
15 minutes

Makes
4 1½-cup servings

Per Serving
Calories: 233
Calories from fat: 34
Total fat: 4 g
Saturated fat: 2 g
Cholesterol: 0 mg
Sodium: 7 mg
Carbohydrates: 50 g
Fiber: 3 g
Sugars: 37 g
Protein: 3 g
Vitamin A: 1% DV
Vitamin C: 2% DV
Calcium: 7% DV
Iron: 8% DV

Almond Butter and Jelly Breakfast Pizza

Pizza for breakfast? Why not! Almonds—high in protein, calcium, and magnesium—are a great way to start the day. By using organic jelly you will avoid pesticides and high fructose corn syrup, a highly refined source of sugar. Get the kids involved in putting this together at the end. It's great fun.

1 cup ground flaxseed

1 cup water

¼ teaspoons salt

2 teaspoons vegetable oil

½ cup of almond butter

½ cup unsweetened jelly of choice

½ cup toasted coconut flakes

2 bananas, sliced

Preheat a skillet to medium-high. Melt oil in skillet.

Put the flaxseed, water, salt, and 1 teaspoon of oil in a mixing bowl and combine.

To make the crust, heat the remaining 1 teaspoon of oil in a nonstick skillet or griddle over medium-high heat. Drop ⅙ of the flaxseed mixture into the skillet, leaving about ½ inch between them and making 6 crusts total. Cook in separate batches if needed. Cook for 3 minutes, until golden. Flip and cook 3 minutes longer.

Remove the pizza crust to a serving platter. Spread the almond butter over the crust as if you were saucing a pizza. Spread the jelly over the nut butter. Top with toasted coconut flakes to look like cheese. Top with sliced banana cut to look like pepperoni.

Free of
casein, corn, dairy, eggs, fish, gluten, soy

Prep time
10 minutes

Total time
20 minutes

Makes
6 servings

Per Serving
Calories: 272
Calories from fat: 72
Total fat: 8 g
Saturated fat: 0 g
Cholesterol: 22 g
Sodium: 27 mg
Carbohydrates: 27 g
Fiber: 7 g
Sugars: 14 g
Protein: 4 g
Vitamin A: 0% DV
Vitamin C: 4% DV
Calcium: 11% DV
Iron: 9% DV

Pecan 'n' Banana Breakfast Bread

Clients are always asking me to help them to consume less carbs. I feel like this is a very healthy way to eat, and this bread is a great way to embrace the low-carb lifestyle. Protein-rich crushed pecans take the place of flour and give this bread a warm, nutty texture that I am sure you and your waistline will love. If you can't find pecans, walnuts would also work well here. Serve the bread with the organic jelly of your choice and a fruit salad for a complete breakfast.

5 cups pecan pieces

Pinch salt

½ teaspoon cinnamon

2 ripe bananas, mashed

½ cup honey or maple syrup

1 tablespoon extra virgin coconut oil

Preheat the oven to 350°F.

Put the pecan pieces in a food processor and process until the nuts resemble the texture of flour. Put the pecan flour in a mixing bowl and add the salt and cinnamon.

In separate bowl, mix the mashed banana with honey. Add to the dry mixture. Add coconut oil and mix thoroughly.

Line an 8 × 4–inch loaf pan with parchment paper. Spread batter evenly into pan.

Bake for 45 minutes. Allow bread to cool, about 15 minutes, before removing it from the pan.

Free of
casein, corn, dairy, eggs, gluten, soy

Prep time
15 minutes

Total time
1 hour

Makes
1 loaf (12 slices)

Per Slice
Calories: 409
Calories from fat: 207
Total fat: 23 g
Saturated fat: 3 g
Cholesterol: 0 mg
Sodium: 27 mg
Carbohydrates: 29 g
Fiber: 6 g
Sugars: 14 g
Protein: 5 g
Vitamin A: 1% DV
Vitamin C: 5% DV
Calcium: 5% DV
Iron: 10% DV

Wonderful Blueberry Walnut Waffles

Blueberries were all the rage in the early 2000s when nutritionists were talking about their high antioxidant content. In addition to their antioxidant power, blueberries also have a low glycemic index, which makes them an acceptable fruit for those with Candida or blood-sugar issues.

3 teaspoons coconut oil, melted

1 cup gluten-free pancake mix

¼ cup puréed sweet potato or jarred baby food

¾ cup frozen blueberries

½ cup walnuts, coarsely chopped

Grease a waffle iron with one teaspoon coconut oil and set on medium-high heat. Put the remaining ingredients in a mixing bowl and blend lightly.

Cook waffles according to manufacturer's direction until golden brown, about 3 minutes.

Serve with maple syrup, jelly, fresh fruit, or cinnamon. Enjoy!

Free of
casein, corn, dairy, eggs, gluten, soy

Prep time
5 minutes

Total time
10 minutes

Makes
4 waffles

Per Waffle (Without Topping)
Calories: 173
Calories from fat: 140
Total fat: 17 g
Saturated fat: 7 g
Cholesterol: 0 mg
Sodium: 5 mg
Carbohydrates: 6 g
Fiber: 2 g
Sugars: 3 g
Protein: 2 g
Vitamin A: 24% DV
Vitamin C: 4% DV
Calcium: 2% DV
Iron: 3% DV

Cranberry Strawberry Breakfast Bars

This recipe is one of my favorite breakfasts. I love the nutty flavor from the almond butter with the sweet tartness of the dried cranberry and the crunch from the brown rice crisp. It's filling, too! One bar keeps me energized for hours afterward. To save on calories you can omit the seeds. This is a gentle-on-your-stomach and an excellent on-the-run bar for those with IBD.

7 cups brown rice cereal

¾ cup dried cranberries

¾ cup dried strawberries

½ cup pumpkin seeds or sunflower seeds

1 teaspoon cinnamon

¾ cup brown rice syrup

¾ cup cashew or almond butter

2 tablespoons butter spread (I like Earth Balance butter spread the best.)

Mix the first five ingredients together in a large mixing bowl.

Put the remaining ingredients in a medium saucepan, over low heat. Stir until well incorporated and heated through. Add to the dry ingredients and coat well.

Using wet hands, spread the cereal mixture onto a 9-inch square baking sheet. Press down firmly, ensuring evenness. Put into the freezer for 1 hour. Slice to make 15 bars. Store in the refrigerator.

Free of
casein, corn, dairy, eggs, gluten, soy

Prep time
1 hour

Total time
65 minutes

Makes
15 bars

Per Bar
Calories: 293
Calories from fat: 108
Total fat: 13 g
Saturated fat: 3 g
Cholesterol: 0 mg
Sodium: 58 mg
Carbohydrates: 41 g
Fiber: 3 g
Sugars: 13 g
Protein: 6 g
Vitamin A: 3% DV
Vitamin C: 10% DV
Calcium: 2% DV
Iron: 11% DV

Pepper and Potato Hash

Who says you can't have hash without eggs? For those egg-intolerant people out there, here is an excellent, filling breakfast hash! The pepper and onion give it sweetness and crunch.

2 pounds red potatoes, peeled and cubed

1 large Vidalia onion, diced

2 green peppers, cut into match sticks

3 tablespoons olive oil

Salt and pepper

Sliced bacon or ham (optional)

Heat the oil in a large skillet over medium-high heat. Add the onion and sauté for 5 minutes. Add pepper and potatoes and continue to sauté, stirring frequently. Cover and cook for about 15 minutes or until potatoes are soft and golden brown.

Continue to add more oil, if necessary. Season with salt and pepper.

Free of
casein, corn, dairy, eggs, fish, gluten, nuts, soy

Prep time
15 minutes

Cook time
15 minutes

Makes
4 servings

Per Serving
Calories: 570
Calories from fat: 156
Total fat: 18 g
Saturated fat: 3 g
Cholesterol: 5 mg
Sodium: 96 mg
Carbohydrates: 96 g
Fiber: 11 g
Sugars: 9 g
Protein: 12 g
Vitamin A: 6% DV
Vitamin C: 184% DV
Calcium: 7% DV
Iron: 25% DV

Groovy Green Eggs and Ham

A little Dr. Seuss for you! You know eating breakfast every day is important and so is eating your vegetables. What better way to do so than with this fun, tasty and, of course, nutritious breakfast starring spinach. I recommend using organic whenever possible, and please use extra care with choosing organic eggs and spinach. It is very important to always choose organic greens, as leafy vegetables are the most heavily pesticide-ridden crops. The eggs will always be more nutritious when organic, making this an important choice.

6 large eggs

10 ounces fresh baby spinach, finely chopped

2 slices of deli ham, diced

Salt and pepper to taste

1 teaspoon olive oil

½ cup toasted pine nuts

12 heaping teaspoons pesto

Cherry tomatoes, diced, for garnish (optional)

Whisk the eggs in a large mixing bowl until frothy.

Fold in the spinach and ham. Season to taste with salt and pepper.

Put the pine nuts in a heavy, small, dry skillet over medium-high heat. Shake and stir until toasted, about 1–2 minutes. Be careful not to burn them. When you can smell their aroma you'll know they are finished. Set aside.

Heat the olive oil in a large skillet over medium heat. Add the eggs and scramble until they are no longer runny.

Plate the eggs and top with pine nuts and pesto.

Free of
casein, corn, gluten, nuts, soy

Prep time
10 minutes

Total time
20 minutes

Makes
4 servings

Per Serving
Calories: 327
Calories from fat: 252
Total fat: 28 g
Saturated fat: 5 g
Cholesterol: 280 mg
Sodium: 127 mg
Carbohydrates: 7 g
Fiber: 1 g
Sugars: 2 g
Protein: 14 g
Vitamin A: 89% DV
Vitamin C: 50% DV
Calcium: 9% DV
Iron: 17% DV

Blissful Breakfast Wrap

This is a great on-the-go recipe. I like to wrap it in parchment paper and eat it on my way to work. If you can't tolerate adzuki beans just eliminate them from the recipe.

½ cup medium salsa
½ cup cooked adzuki beans
Handful baby spinach
4 eggs
4 gluten-free brown rice tortillas

Possible toppings:
Grated raw cheddar cheese or soy substitute
Chopped scallions
Chopped parsley or cilantro
Tofu or almond-milk cheese
Sliced avocado
Taco sauce

Free of
casein, corn, dairy, fish, gluten, nuts, soy

Prep time
5 minutes

Total time
20 minutes

Makes
2 servings

Per Serving (Without Toppings)
Calories: 322
Calories from fat: 80
Total fat: 9 g
Saturated fat: 2 g
Cholesterol: 257 g
Sodium: 539 mg
Carbohydrates: 50 g
Fiber: 2 g
Sugars: 2 g
Protein: 11 g
Vitamin A: 21% DV
Vitamin C: 16% DV
Calcium: 5% DV
Iron: 16% DV

Heat the salsa and adzuki beans in a large non-stick skillet over medium heat for 5 minutes. Add the spinach and stir to incorporate.

Put the spinach mixture to one side. Crack eggs into the pan and cook 3–5 minutes to desired firmness, whether sunny side up or scrambled.

Meanwhile, toast the tortillas in a toaster oven until soft.

Place the sandwich wraps side by side on a cutting board and slide half of the eggs and spinach mixture onto each one. Gather the wrap and tuck the filling under the tortilla and roll like a cigar. Garnish with your choice of toppings.

Good Morning Buckwheat

Contrary to its name, buckwheat, also known as kasha, actually does not contain wheat. It is part of the rhubarb family of plants. I love buckwheat because it is high in protein, making it an ideal grain for weight loss and endurance. It is gluten free, of course, so it's also gentle on sensitive tummies.

1 cup buckwheat, cooked according to package instructions

1 apple, grated

½ cup shredded carrots

2 tablespoons almond or cashew butter

1 teaspoon cinnamon

1 teaspoon vanilla

1 teaspoon maple syrup

¼ cup chopped cashews or almonds

Free of
casein, corn, dairy, eggs, fish, gluten, soy

Prep time
5 minutes

Total time
45 minutes

Makes
2 servings

Per Serving
Calories: 120
Calories from fat: 23
Total fat: 3 g
Saturated fat: 1 g
Cholesterol: 0 mg
Sodium: 23 mg
Carbohydrates: 20 g
Fiber: 3.5 g
Sugars: 2.5 g
Protein: 4 g
Vitamin A: 16% DV
Vitamin C: 3% DV
Calcium: 5% DV
Iron: 4% DV

Cook the buckwheat according to package directions. Pour buckwheat into a mixing bowl and add the apple and carrots.

In a small bowl mix the nut butter with 2 tablespoons of hot water. Blend with fork until creamy like a sauce. If needed, add a bit more water, but mixture should not be too runny.

Pour the blended butter over buckwheat mixture. Sprinkle with cinnamon, vanilla, and maple syrup. Sprinkle crushed nuts on top.

Time-saving tip: Make the buckwheat the night before for a dinner dish and remove a cup for breakfast the next day. Warm it in the microwave. With a splash of olive oil, buckwheat will keep well for 3 or 4 days in the refrigerator.

Potato, Bacon, and Arugula Hash

This hash is enhanced with smoky bacon and spicy arugula. It is a great way to start the day off! You can't go wrong with greens and healthy proteins in the morning. If you are having a flare-up, cook the greens until they are very soft.

1 onion, diced

2 garlic gloves, chopped

½ red pepper, diced

3 tablespoons olive oil

4 baby red potatoes, peeled and diced

3 cups arugula

4 strips of turkey bacon

8 grape tomatoes, diced

Salt and pepper to taste

Sauté the onions, garlic, and red pepper in the olive oil for 5 minutes. Add the potatoes and cook for 10 minutes, covered, stirring occasionally.

While the potatoes are cooking, cut the turkey bacon into bite-size pieces with kitchen shears. Cook the bacon in a separate, small pan until browned and crisp. Remove with a slotted spoon and blot with a paper towel.

Stir the arugula into the potatoes until it is wilted. Add the tomatoes and bring to a simmer. Cook uncovered for 5 minutes.

Top with the turkey bacon and season to taste.

Free of
casein, corn, dairy, eggs, fish, gluten, nuts, soy

Prep time
15 minutes

Total time
35 minutes

Makes
2 servings

Per Serving
Calories: 414
Calories from fat: 121
Total fat: 14 g
Saturated fat: 2 g
Cholesterol: 13 g
Sodium: 197 mg
Carbohydrates: 66 g
Fiber: 8 g
Sugars: 7 g
Protein: 10 g
Vitamin A: 32% DV
Vitamin C: 149% DV
Calcium: 7% DV
Iron: 18% DV

For people with inflammatory bowel disease (IBD), a nutritious drink is soothing medicine. The smoothie recipes in this section are particularly helpful when your insides are acting up. I highly recommend putting yourself on a smoothie/soup regime to help optimize nutrition when you are flaring up. Since these types of foods are puréed, they require significantly less effort to breakdown. When I was in the hospital during a flare-up, a nurse recommended that I eat baby food as a sort of modified bowel rest. I found this worked very well, and I began suggesting it to clients.

Even though baby food made me feel better, I didn't find the idea terribly appealing. I decided there must be a better way, so I developed the smoothie recipes found in this book. Try them until you're feeling better. Then you can gradually begin to introduce more solid, substantial foods.

Because dehydration plays a substantial role in flare-ups for most with inflammatory bowel disease, it is important to choose foods that assist the body in restoring electrolyte balances. Sugary sports drinks are not the best option because they contain artificial flavors, colors, and excessive amounts of sugar.

The beverages featured in this section are intended to change up the same old, same old and give you inspiration for trying new foods. Water should still be your primary source of hydration, along with coconut water. Coconut water is crucial, as it can restore electrolyte imbalance much more effectively than sports drinks; since it is from a natural source, your body can break down the nutrients in it more easily than those found in artificial electrolyte drinks. Coconut water contains potassium, sodium, and magnesium, three important electrolytes.[1]

If you are intolerant of dairy, you will find several dairy-free substitutions that you can make at home. With these tasty recipes, you will not miss dairy ever again. Additionally, this section is home to some amazingly refreshing smoothie recipes, such as my prized Strawberry Cranberry Smoothie (see page 164). This section is important for you if you are experiencing a flare-up. By consuming smoothies and giving your bowels a rest, you are significantly helping the digestive tract heal while still providing your body with essential nutrients and minerals. Smoothies are a great alternative to a standard breakfast.

Strawberry Cranberry Smoothie

Healthy and fast, this smoothie is out of this world. Slightly tart from the cranberry and kissed with a hint of sweetness from the vanilla and strawberry, this morning pick-me-up is sure to please your taste buds.

1 cup unsweetened coconut milk, coconut water, or soy French vanilla yogurt
1 cup cranberry juice
1 16-ounce package frozen strawberries

Place all the ingredients into a blender and purée for about 3 minutes. Serve and enjoy!

Free of
casein, corn, dairy, eggs, fish, gluten, nuts, soy

Prep time
10 minutes

Total time
13 minutes

Makes
2 servings

Per Serving
Calories: 244
Calories from fat: 32
Total fat: 3.5 g
Saturated fat: 2.5 g
Cholesterol: 0 mg
Sodium: 7 mg
Carbohydrates: 70 g
Fiber: 10 g
Sugars: 6 g
Protein: 2.5 g
Vitamin A: 2% DV
Vitamin C: 184% DV
Calcium: 25% DV
Iron: 10% DV

Coconut Water Coolada

This is one of my favorite health-restoring drinks, as it is excellent for replenishing minerals and electrolytes, which is especially important during or after a flare-up. The ginger works quite well to reduce nausea. This drink is anti-inflammatory, making it good for restoring and maintaining optimum digestive health. Take advantage of it when you find fresh papayas in the market.

2 17-ounce containers coconut water (coconut water is available in most grocery stores or you can purchase it online)

1 medium papaya, very ripe

1-inch piece gingerroot, peeled and coarsely chopped

2 tablespoons honey (raw honey is preferable because it still has its enzymes intact, is not processed, and is higher in nutrients)

Place all the ingredients into blender and purée until smooth, about 2 minutes.

Serve iced or at room temperature.

Free of
casein, corn, dairy, eggs, fish, gluten, nuts, soy

Prep time
5 minutes

Total time
10 minutes

Makes
2 servings

Per Serving
Calories: 73
Calories from fat: 0
Total fat: 0 g
Cholesterol: 0 mg
Sodium: 66 mg
Carbohydrates: 18 g
Fiber: 2 g
Sugars: 14 g
Protein: 1 g
Vitamin A: 15% DV
Vitamin C: 75% DV
Calcium: 3% DV
Iron: 2% DV

Peachy-Keen Smoothie

When I make Grilled Peaches (see page 178) I make an extra batch so I can have this smoothie the next day. They keep well refrigerated.

3 cups almond milk
1 medium or large ripe banana
1 recipe Grilled Peaches, cooled (Grilled Peaches can be made ahead of time, see recipe on page 178)

Place all the ingredients in a blender and purée for 1–2 minutes, until all is incorporated.

Serve warm in the winter and chilled in the summer.

Free of
casein, corn, dairy, eggs, gluten, soy

Prep time
15 minutes

Total time
20 minutes

Makes
4 servings

Per Serving
Calories: 94
Calories from fat: 11
Total fat: 1 g
Saturated fat: 0 g
Cholesterol: 0 mg
Sodium: 46 mg
Carbohydrates: 22 g
Fiber: 3 g
Sugars: 14 g
Protein: 2 g
Vitamin A: 9% DV
Vitamin C: 18% DV
Calcium: 8% DV
Iron: 3% DV

Pumped-Up Piña Colada Smoothie

This smoothie is ideal for maintaining digestive health. It is also a great choice when your stomach is not feeling 100 percent. Pineapple naturally contains bromelain, a digestive enzyme that can be very beneficial for those with Crohn's disease. Coconut is well known for its soothing, anti-inflammatory properties in the intestine. Please choose organic coconuts and coconut milk, as they are more nutrient-dense and lack potentially harmful pesticides and chemicals.

1 14.5-ounce can coconut milk
1 cup chopped fresh pineapple or 1 can crushed
   pineapple with juice
1 fresh peeled banana, frozen overnight

Place all the ingredients in a blender and purée for about 3 minutes.

Serve and enjoy!

Free of
casein, corn, dairy, eggs, fish, gluten, nuts, soy

Prep time
10 minutes

Total time
13 minutes

Makes
2 8-ounce glasses

Per Serving
Calories: 209
Calories from fat: 122
Total fat: 15 g
Saturated fat: 13 g
Cholesterol: 0 mg
Sodium: 10 mg
Carbohydrates: 22 g
Fiber: 3 g
Sugars: 13 g
Protein: 2 g
Vitamin A: 1% DV
Vitamin C: 44% DV
Calcium: 2% DV
Iron: 7% DV

Homemade Vanilla Almond Milk

The wonderfully nutty, sweet taste of almond milk is an excellent choice for people who are intolerant of dairy—and it has even more calcium than milk! This recipe makes a large batch and will keep well in the refrigerator for three days. Please use organic almonds, as regular almonds are on the Environmental Working Group's Dirty Dozen list as they can contain high levels of pesticide residues. Chemicals such as these can potentially irritate someone with IBD more than they would someone else.

1 cup almonds, soaked in water overnight in the refrigerator and rinsed
3 cups filtered water
Seeds from 1 vanilla bean
5 soft, pitted dates
¼ cup agave nectar
½ cup brown rice syrup or agave nectar

Put the soaked almonds and the water in a blender and purée until smooth, about 2 minutes. Strain mixture into a large bowl. Refrigerate the almond pulp for later use.

Return the strained milk to the blender and add the vanilla beans, dates, and rice syrup/agave until smooth. Shake well before serving.

Variation: Blend in a banana and use a pinch of nutmeg to make a festive raw nog.

Free of
casein, corn, dairy, eggs, fish, gluten, soy

Prep time
10 minutes

Total time
10 minutes

Makes
12 servings

Per Serving
Calories: 98
Calories from fat: 51
Total fat: 6 g
Saturated fat: 0 g
Cholesterol: 0 mg
Sodium: 3 mg
Carbohydrates: 10 g
Fiber: 2 g
Sugars: 7 g
Protein: 3 g
Vitamin A: 0% DV
Vitamin C: 0% DV
Calcium: 3% DV
Iron: 3% DV

Christie's Groovy Green Machine Juice

This is my take on Naked brand smoothie drinks, which I love. They are high in nutrition and taste great, and they incorporate fruits, vegetables, and even protein. They are excellent for a flare-up since they contain fruit that is already broken down, thereby making them more gentle. I always use organic apples, as conventional apples are also on the EWG Dirty Dozen list of pesticide-laden foods.

1 cup raw spinach, tightly packed

2 celery stalks, cut into thirds

3 carrots, peeled

2 gala apples

2 kiwis

Juice of one lemon

2 teaspoons "green powder" (my favorite, Garden of Life Perfect Food, can be purchased online at http://www.gardenoflife.com)

Put the vegetables, fruit, and lemon juice in a juicer and process until smooth, about 5 minutes. Once the juice is completed, you can stir in the green powder. Chill, or enjoy at room temperature.

Free of
casein, corn, dairy, eggs, gluten, nuts, soy

Prep time
10 minutes

Total time
25 minutes

Makes
2 servings

Per Serving
Calories: 97
Calories from fat: 6
Total fat: less than 1 g
Saturated fat: 0 g
Cholesterol: 0 mg
Sodium: 73 mg
Carbohydrates: 24 g
Fiber: 4 g
Sugars: 13 g
Protein: 3 g
Vitamin A: 107% DV
Vitamin C: 179% DV
Calcium: 9% DV
Iron: 11% DV

Very Vanilla Rice Milk

This drink is excellent for restoring hydration after a bout with diarrhea. For decades, doctors have been recommending brown rice to treat the dehydration that accompanies dysentery. Make sure the water is hot, as cold water and rice will not mix. The best way to make this is immediately after preparing the rice, while it is still hot.

1 cup cooked short-grain brown rice
4 cups simmering-hot filtered water
2 teaspoons vanilla extract

Put all the ingredients in a blender and process until smooth. Allow the mixture to sit for 30 minutes.

Pour the mixture into a pitcher draped with cheesecloth to collect the sediment.

Alternative: For a smoother milk, re-cook left-over rice with the filtered water until it's very soft. Add a pinch of salt and some brown rice syrup or agave nectar to taste. You can also try soaked, blanched almonds or other nuts (use the same measurements as for the rice and blend until smooth).

Free of
casein, corn, dairy, eggs, fish, gluten, nuts, soy

Prep time
10 minutes

Total time
45–60 minutes

Makes
4 servings

Per Serving
Calories: 55
Calories from fat: 3
Total fat: less than 1 g
Saturated fat: 0 g
Cholesterol: 0 mg
Sodium: 0 mg
Carbohydrates: 11 g
Fiber: 1 g
Sugars: 0 g
Protein: 1 g
Vitamin A: 0% DV
Vitamin C: 0% DV
Calcium: 0% DV
Iron: 1% DV

Simple Watermelon Chiller

This recipe makes for excellent ice pops. Simply pour into a popsicle/ice pop mold and freeze. It makes a refreshing treat! Watermelon is very hydrating and is great during a flare-up, especially if you have lost electrolytes. This is a perfect sweet that will also be gentle on your sensitive stomach!

3 cups coarsely chopped watermelon without
    seeds
Juice of one lemon

Put the watermelon and lemon juice in a blender on liquefy mode and process about 2–3 minutes, until smooth.

Serve chilled.

Free of
casein, corn, dairy, eggs, fish, gluten, nuts, soy

Prep time
5 minutes

Total time
8 minutes

Makes
2 servings

Per Serving
Calories: 38
Calories from fat: 1
Total fat: less than 1 g
Saturated fat: 0 g
Cholesterol: 0 mg
Sodium: 1 mg
Carbohydrates: 10 g
Fiber: 1 g
Sugars: 7 g
Protein: 1 g
Vitamin A: 13% DV
Vitamin C: 25% DV
Calcium: 1% DV
Iron: 2% DV

Pumpkin Pie Healthy Egg Cream

This is an excellent recipe for you "Brooklynites" out there. It's just like the ones you are used to from the local deli, but with a healthy pumpkin twist.

1 large free-range egg
2 cups soy, rice, or almond milk
½ cup coconut oil
2 tablespoons pure maple syrup
1 teaspoon vanilla
½ teaspoon pumpkin pie spice

Place all the ingredients into a container or blender with a tight-fitting lid and either shake or blend until smooth and thick. Chill for at least 2 hours before serving.

Variation: Substitute 1 cup of sparkling water for 1 cup of the milk. This creates a more bubbly treat.

Free of
casein, corn, dairy, eggs, fish, gluten, nuts, soy

Prep time
N/A

Total time
2 hours, unattended

Makes about
3 1-cup servings

Per Serving
Calories: 363
Calories from fat: 135
Total fat: 15 g
Saturated fat: 4 g
Cholesterol: 257 g
Sodium: 131 mg
Carbohydrates: 8 mg
Fiber: 0 g
Sugars: 6 g
Protein: 8 g
Vitamin A: 8% DV
Vitamin C: 0% DV
Calcium: 11% DV
Iron: 8% DV

Gentle Ginger Peppermint Chiller

Consider this drink a staple to help combat a flare-up.

1 pound fresh gingerroot, peeled and grated
6 cups water
1 peppermint tea bag
Juice of 2 limes
Maple syrup or agave nectar to taste

Put the ginger, water, and tea bag in a large saucepan and bring to a boil. Simmer for 5 minutes.

Strain the liquid through a fine mesh sieve and add the lime juice and sweetener and stir until dissolved. Refrigerate for 1 day before serving.

Free of
casein, corn, dairy, fish, gluten, nuts, soy

Prep time
10 minutes

Total time
1 day, unattended

Makes
8 servings

Per Serving
Calories: 14
Calories from fat: 0
Total fat: 0 g
Saturated fat: 0 g
Cholesterol: 0 mg
Sodium: 1 mg
Carbohydrates: 4 g
Fiber: 0 g
Sugars: 2 g
Protein: 0 g
Vitamin A: 0% DV
Vitamin C: 7% DV
Calcium: 0% DV
Iron: 0% DV

Pineapple Cherry-licious Explosion

Pineapples and cherries are a great combination that you rarely see, except maybe on your grandmother's Christmas ham. I think it is a pairing of flavors that is underutilized. This drink is designed to change that. But there is a surprise: The flavor comes from the pineapple core, not the flesh. This recipe has been modified from its original version and was inspired by the Institute for Integrative Nutrition.

1 ripe pineapple
2 limes, thinly sliced
3 whole cloves
4 slices peeled ginger root, crushed
2 pints boiling water
Agave nectar to taste (optional)
5 fresh bing cherries, pitted and finely chopped
Lime slices for garnish

Peel the pineapple, and cut the peel into large chunks. Reserve the flesh for use in another dish. Place the pineapple peel, ginger, limes, and cloves in a large bowl. Pour the boiling water over the mixture, cover, and steep for 24 hours.

Discard the pineapple peel, limes, and cloves, and strain the liquid through a piece of cheesecloth into a drink container. Add agave nectar to taste. Serve chilled with a garnish of chopped cherries and lime.

Free of
casein, corn, dairy, eggs, gluten, nuts, soy

Prep time
10 minutes

Total time
24 hours, unattended

Makes
6 servings

Per Serving
Calories: 47
Calories from fat: 1
Total fat: less than 1 g
Saturated fat: 0 g
Cholesterol: 0 mg
Sodium: 1 mg
Carbohydrates: 13 g
Fiber: 1 g
Sugars: 9 g
Protein: 0 g
Vitamin A: 2% DV
Vitamin C: 45% DV
Calcium: 1% DV
Iron: 1% DV

APPETIZERS and SNACK FOODS

Eating small meals can be ideal for those with IBD, especially if you don't usually have a huge appetite. So I'd like to include some appetizers and finger foods for you to check out during those times that you don't want to overinduldge and just need a small pick-me-up.

These appetizers are excellent for parties as well, and all have been modified with your special digestive system in mind!

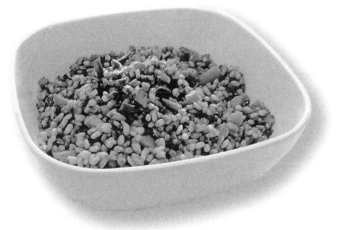

Falafel Nuggets with Tomato Sauce

This recipe comes from my dear friend Penny Fellas. She is an expert in all things Greek and was kind enough to share this favorite with me. It can be served with a side of brown rice and steamed squash. If you can't tolerate tomato sauce, try Greek yogurt or simply sprinkle the nuggets with some olive oil and lemon juice to add some extra flavor. This dish is moderately anti-inflammatory.

For the falafel:

2 15-ounce cans chickpeas

½ cup rice flour

½ cup chopped fresh parsley

½ chopped onion

1 tablespoon ground flaxseed mixed in 3 tablespoons warm water

2 teaspoons cumin

½ teaspoon red pepper

For the sauce:

2½ cups tomato sauce

⅓ cup tomato paste

2 tablespoons ascorbic acid crystals (found in health-food store) or lemon juice, if tolerated

2 teaspoons honey

1 teaspoon onion powder

½ teaspoon salt

Small handful fresh parsley, chopped

2 basil leaves, chopped

Free of
casein, corn, dairy, eggs, fish, gluten

Prep time
15 minutes

Total time
1 hour

Makes
12 servings

Per Serving
Calories: 346
Calories from fat: 46
Total fat: 5 g
Saturated fat: 1 g
Cholesterol: 0 mg
Sodium: 536 mg
Carbohydrates: 69 g
Fiber: 12 g
Sugar: 19 g
Protein: 12 g
Vitamin A: 41% DV
Vitamin C: 54% DV
Calcium: 14% DV
Iron: 39% DV

Preheat oven to 400°F.

Put all the ingredients for the falafel in a food processor and pulse until well combined. Form the mixture into 1-inch balls. You should have about 12–15 balls. Line the balls on a baking sheet sprayed with olive oil or lined with parchment paper.

Combine all the sauce ingredients in a medium sauce pan over medium heat. Bring to a simmer and cook for 20 minutes.

Bake the falafel for 10 minutes, or until golden brown. Serve with sauce on the side for dipping.

Grilled Peaches

I love making this recipe in the summer, when peaches are at the peak of season. It is simple and fast, and is a wonderful and sweet way to end to your favorite barbeque.

1 dozen peaches, cut in half, pitted
3 tablespoons agave nectar
1 teaspoon lemon juice
1 teaspoon cinnamon
Pinch of allspice

Preheat outdoor grill or grill pan to medium-high or high heat.

Cut the peaches in half vertically and remove pits. Put the peaches in a large bowl and set aside.

Pour the remaining ingredients over the peaches and coat well.

Put the peaches on grilling pan over preheated outdoor grill set on high.

Grill for 5 minutes on each side, or until you have some grill marks.

Serve peaches over coconut yogurt with blueberries or granola.

Free of
casein, corn, dairy, eggs, fish, gluten

Prep time
10 minutes

Total time
15 minutes

Makes
6 servings

Per Serving
Calories: 157
Calories from fat: 8
Total fat: 1 g
Saturated Fat: 0 g
Cholesterol: 1 mg
Sodium: 1 mg
Carbohydrates: 41 g
Fiber: 7 g
Sugar: 12 g
Protein: 3 g
Vitamin A: 23% DV
Vitamin C: 45% DV
Calcium: 5% DV
Iron: 6% DV

Brown Rice Quesadillas

Who doesn't love a quesadilla? If you are gluten intolerant, these are a real treat, especially if you have not yet discovered brown-rice wraps. I find they are just as good, if not better than, the traditional wheat-flour version.

1 cup commercial salsa
½ cup cooked black beans (pinto or navy beans can be substituted)
2 avocados, peeled and sliced
2 brown-rice sandwich wraps

Combine the salsa, avocado, and beans in a mixing bowl.

Heat a large skillet to medium-high. Place one wrap in the skillet. Spread half the avocado filling all over the wrap, as if you were spreading sauce on a pizza, keeping it clear of the outer ½ inch of the wrap.

Place another wrap on top of the first. Using your fingers, carefully press together the edges of the wraps. Cook for about 5 minutes.

Using a spatula, flip the wrap. Cook for about 4 minutes, or until crispy and brown on the outside.

Using a pizza cutter, slice each quesadilla in half, and then cut the halves in half. Cut the halves in half again so you have 8 slices total. Serve with extra salsa on top, if desired.

Free of
casein, corn, dairy, eggs, fish, gluten

Prep time
5 minutes

Total time
15 minutes

Makes
4 servings

Per Serving
Calories: 296
Calories from fat: 112
Total fat: 13 g
Saturated fat: 2 g
Cholesterol: 0 mg
Sodium: 214 mg
Carbohydrates: 39 g
Fiber: 11 g
Sugar: 4 g
Protein: 9 g
Vitamin A: 5% DV
Vitamin C: 39% DV
Calcium: 4% DV
Iron: 12% DV

Buttery Banana Cupcakes

If you like bananas, you will really enjoy this moist, dense, creamy cupcake. Enjoy!

2 large ripe bananas, broken into pieces

½ cup coconut oil

½ cup water

½ cup agave nectar

1 teaspoon almond extract

⅛ teaspoon ground flaxseed

1¾ cups gluten-free flour

1 tablespoon baking powder

1 teaspoon pumpkin pie spice

½ teaspoon xanthan gum

½ teaspoon salt

Preheat oven to 350°F.

Put the bananas in the bowl of an electric mixer. Add the oil, water, agave, almond extract, and flaxseed, and beat for 1 minute.

In a small bowl, combine the flour, baking powder, pumpkin pie spice, xanthan, and salt. Add to the banana mixture. Beat for 1 minute on low or until batter is smooth.

Line the tins of a 12-muffin tin with muffin-tin liners. Pour the batter into the tins. Bake for 1 hour, or until golden brown and a toothpick inserted in a muffin comes out clean. Cool before removing from pan.

Free of
casein, corn, dairy, eggs, fish, gluten

Prep time
10 minutes

Total time
70 minutes

Makes
1 dozen cupcakes

Per Serving
Calories: 347
Calories from fat: 114
Total fat: 13 g
Saturated fat: 10 g
Cholesterol: 0 mg
Sodium: 210 mg
Carbohydrates: 56 g
Fiber: 4 g
Sugar: 12 g
Protein: 4 g
Vitamin A: 1% DV
Vitamin C: 11% DV
Calcium: 2% DV
Iron: 7% DV

Apple Cinnamon Granola

Cinnamon is great way to quell a sugar craving because it is sweet. This granola mix is a great between-meal snack, especially when you need an energy boost. It also stays fresh for a long time.

4 cups quinoa flakes
1 cup finely chopped pecans
½ cup grated or flaked coconut
½ cup sesame seeds
¾ teaspoon salt
1 teaspoon cinnamon
½ cup coconut oil
½ cup raw honey
1 teaspoon vanilla
½ pound dried apples, chopped

Preheat oven to 350°F.

In a large bowl combine the quinoa, nuts, coconut, sesame seeds, cinnamon, and salt.

Put the oil, honey, and vanilla in a medium sauce over low heat for 5 minutes. Add to the quinoa mixture and toss to coat evenly. Spread out on a cookie sheet sprayed with olive oil or lined with parchment.

Bake for 20 minutes. Remove from the oven and mix in the dried apple pieces. Store in an airtight container.

Free of
casein, corn, dairy, eggs, fish, gluten

Prep time
10 minutes

Total time
30 minutes

Makes about
6 1-cup servings

Per Serving
Calories: 350
Calories from fat: 137
Total Fat: 16 g
Saturated fat: 5 g
Cholesterol: 0 mg
Sodium: 15 mg
Carbohydrates: 46 g
Fiber: 6 g
Sugar: 13 g
Protein: 9 g
Vitamin A: 0% DV
Vitamin C: 1% DV
Calcium: 11% DV
Iron: 20% DV

Sweet Potato Muffins

These muffins are more savory than sweet—they will surprise you. Serve them along with dinner or as accompaniment to a Sunday brunch.

2 cups gluten-free baking mix
Pinch of salt
1 tablespoon flaxseed mixed with 3 teaspoons hot water
1 cup grated sweet potato
½ cup parsley, finely chopped
1 cup coconut milk
1 teaspoon pumpkin pie spice

Preheat oven to 325°F.

Mix the flour and salt in a bowl by hand or using an electric mixer. Add the flaxseed/water mixture, sweet potatoes, and parsley.

Mix lightly, gradually adding the milk. The consistency should be lumpy, so don't mix too much! Add the pumpkin pie spice.

Spoon the batter into a lightly oiled muffin tray. Bake for 12–15 minutes or until a fork inserted into the middle comes out clean.

Remove and allow to set for 10 minutes before serving.

Free of
casein, corn, dairy, eggs, fish, gluten

Prep time
5 minutes

Total time
20 minutes

Makes
12 muffins

Per Muffin
Calories: 122
Calories from fat: 17
Total fat: 2 g
Saturated fat: 1 g
Cholesterol: 0 mg
Sodium: 12 mg
Carbohydrates: 24 g
Fiber: 2 g
Sugar: 1 g
Protein: 2 g
Vitamin A: 37% DV
Vitamin C: 6% DV
Calcium: 3% DV
Iron: 5% DV

I have found both personally and professionally that soup is an extremely valuable resource for those with IBD. If you are flaring-up, I highly recommend it. It's easy to prepare, economical, and, above all, extremely nutrient dense and easy to breakdown. It is helpful to introduce soups and smoothies as a way to rest your bowels. This will allow for your stomach to have a "break" from assimilating harder-to-digest, more-solid foods.

20-Minute Tomato Soup

This soup is a quick solution for dinner at the end of a hectic day. For a family of four, it will provide leftovers for lunch the next day. This dish is mildly anti-inflammatory.

1 medium onion, diced
1 cup diced carrots
3 tablespoons olive oil
1 cup chopped spinach
2 14-ounce cans tomato soup
1 cup cooked brown rice
8 basil leaves, shredded
Salt and pepper to taste
½ cup chopped toasted walnuts (optional)

In a large soup pot, sauté the onions and carrots in the olive oil for 5 minutes, until soft. Add the spinach and cook 1 more minute. Add tomato soup, basil, and brown rice. Serve topped with toasted walnuts for a Parmesan cheese–like topping.

Free of
casein, corn, dairy, eggs, fish, gluten

Prep time
10 minutes

Total time
20 minutes

Makes
8 servings

Per Serving
Calories: 127
Calories from fat: 84
Total fat: 10 g
Saturated fat: 1 g
Cholesterol: 0 mg
Sodium: 122 mg
Carbohydrates: 8 g
Fiber: 2 g
Sugar: 2 g
Protein: 2 g
Vitamin A: 14% DV
Vitamin C: 25% DV
Calcium: 2% DV
Iron: 3% DV

Mom's Classic Chicken Soup

There's nothing like Mom's homemade chicken soup. It's so nutrient rich that I serve it as a first course on Sundays. This dish is mildly anti-inflammatory.

1 5-pound chicken
1 large onion, diced
1 cup diced celery
1 cup diced carrots
1 cup chopped parsnips
1 handful parsley, chopped
1 tablespoon salt
Salt and pepper to taste (optional)

Put the chicken in a large soup pot and cover generously with filtered water. Add the salt and bring to a simmer over medium-high heat. Add the onions, celery, carrots, and parsnips.

Cover and cook gently stirring occasionally, until chicken is tender, about 2 or 3 hours.

When the soup cools, remove the chicken and slice. Skim the fat with a mesh strainer and discard. Remove the skin from the chicken and discard. Cut the chicken into ½-inch pieces. If desired, add cooked brown rice or brown rice noodles. Bring back to a simmer. Season with salt and pepper to taste.

Free of
casein, corn, dairy, eggs, fish, gluten

Prep time
30 minutes

Total time
4½ hours or more

Makes
12 servings

Per Serving
Calories: 198
Calories from fat: 93
Total fat: 10 g
Saturated fat: 3 g
Cholesterol: 66 mg
Sodium: 81 mg
Carbohydrates: 4 g
Fiber: 1 g
Sugar: 2 g
Protein: 21 g
Vitamin A: 23% DV
Vitamin C: 17% DV
Calcium: 3% DV
Iron: 8% DV

Nourishing Potato Soup

Potatoes are a valuable starch for those with IBD. They are easier to metabolize than most grains and make a hearty addition to soups by adding a thick, creamy texture.

1 large onion, diced
1 small handful fresh parsley, chopped
2 celery stalks, diced
2 tablespoons olive oil
6 red potatoes, about 1 pound, diced
2 large sweet potatoes, about 1 pound, diced
1½ cups filtered water
1 teaspoon salt
Pinch white pepper
1 cup rice milk
1 teaspoon fresh dill, chopped

Free of
casein, corn, dairy, eggs, fish, gluten

Prep time
15 minutes

Total time
45 minutes

Makes
6 servings

Per Serving
Calories: 227
Calories from fat: 56
Total fat: 6 g
Saturated fat: 1 g
Cholesterol: 0 mg
Sodium: 143 mg
Carbohydrates: 110 g
Fiber: 14 g
Sugar: 13 g
Protein: 12 g
Vitamin A: 476% DV
Vitamin C: 102% DV
Calcium: 13% DV
Iron: 29% DV

In a soup pot, sauté the onions, celery, and parsley in the olive oil for 5 minutes, stirring frequently.

Add the potatoes, water, and salt and pepper to taste. Cover and cook 20 minutes, or until the potatoes are soft.

Using a ladle, blend half the soup in a blender or food processor until smooth. Return the soup to the pot. Add the rice milk. For a creamier consistency, blend all of the soup. Garnish with dill and serve.

Un-French Onion Soup

When I go out to eat, I always tell the wait staff to remove the "French" from my onion soup, since I don't eat the bread or cheese. This dish is mildly anti-inflammatory.

4 medium-large onions, peeled and cut in half

4 teaspoons oil, sesame or olive

4 cups beef broth

4 slices gluten-free French bread or rice bread

4 tablespoons gluten-free tamari

Heat the oil in a large soup pot. When hot, sauté the onions until they start to brown, about 3–5 minutes. Add the broth and bring to boil. Lower the heat and simmer for 20 minutes.

Add the tamari and simmer 3 minutes longer.

Cut the bread into ¼-inch think slices. Toast in toaster oven until slightly browned, about 4 minutes.

Pour the soup into onion soup bowls and float the bread on top.

Free of
casein, corn, dairy, eggs, fish, gluten

Prep time
5 minutes

Total time
35 minutes

Makes
4 servings

Per Serving
Calories: 21
Calories from fat: 11
Total fat: 1 g
Saturated fat: 0 g
Cholesterol: 0 mg
Sodium: 460 mg
Carbohydrates: 2 g
Fiber: 0 g
Sugar: 1 g
Protein: 1 g
Vitamin A: 0% DV
Vitamin C: 2% DV
Calcium: 1% DV
Iron: 1% DV

Many nutritionists believe that people with IBD should avoid beans because they are too hard to digest. However, if they are prepared properly and eaten in combination with other healthy foods, they can be a welcome addition to your diet.

Beans are notorious for producing gas. This is because beans contain a high concentration of trisaccharides, chemical compounds that when broken down into sugar can cause gas and inflammation. This can cause a lot of digestive turmoil, even in healthy people. For those with IBD, studies show trisaccharides can also make you irritable and interfere with clear thinking.

However, not all beans are equally troublesome. The easiest to digest are lentils, peas, mung beans, and kidney beans. If you find you have trouble eating beans, stick with these varieties and only consume them in small quantities. Start with eating just a few tablespoons at a time, and work your way up to increase your tolerance level. You'll know when too much is too much!

Beans belong in a healthy diet because they have many proven curative powers, most notably the ability to help reduce cholesterol. They also have some advantages for people with IBS. For example, one study found that peas help stop constipation and vomiting. The best way to make beans more digestible is to eat them with dark-green leafy vegetables or seaweed.

The beans that are the most difficult to digest are lima, kidney, pinto, garbanzo, and navy beans. Eat them no more than once or twice a month. Avoid *all* types during a flare-up, as they will make your symptoms worse. Once the situation subsides, you can reintroduce them to your diet gradually.

Creamy Coconut Adzuki Beans

This recipe was inspired by the Institute for Integrative Nutrition. Adzuki beans are known to be one of the most easily digestible and nutritious beans.

1 cup dried adzuki beans

2 tablespoons olive oil

1 pound butternut squash, peeled, cleaned, and diced

1 clove garlic, minced

2 red onions, diced

1 15-ounce can coconut milk

1 teaspoon curry powder

2 teaspoons raisins or dried cranberry

1 red pepper, diced

½ cup halved grapes

Rinse the adzuki beans and put in a large pot. Cover generously with water. Bring the beans to a boil over high heat. Reduce the heat, and simmer, uncovered, until soft, about 30 minutes. Drain.

Heat the oil in a large skillet. Add the squash and garlic and then stir-fry for 3–5 minutes.

Add red pepper, raisins, curry powder, and drained adzuki beans. Add the coconut milk and bring to a simmer. Lower the heat, cover, and cook for 20 minutes. Garnish with grapes and serve.

Free of
casein, corn, dairy, eggs, fish, gluten, nuts

Prep time
10 minutes

Total time
40 minutes

Makes
6 servings

Per Serving
Calories: 331
Calories from fat: 48
Total fat: 5 g
Saturated fat: 2 g
Cholesterol: 0 mg
Sodium: 175 mg
Carbohydrates: 68 g
Fiber: 5 g
Sugars: 10 g
Protein: 5 g
Vitamin A: 175% DV
Vitamin C: 116% DV
Calcium: 11% DV
Iron: 14% DV

Roasted Garlic Hummus

Hummus seems to have become more and more popular over the past few years. Chickpeas are relatively simple to digest and offer a creamy and smoky complement to any cracker or crudités platter.

1 head garlic, stem removed

2 tablespoons olive oil

2 cups canned chickpeas

½ red pepper, seeded

3 tablespoons tahini

½ teaspoon salt

½ teaspoon pepper

½ teaspoon cumin

2 tablespoons lemon juice

½ cup or more water

Preheat oven to 450°F.

Put the unpeeled garlic head on a large piece of aluminum foil. Cover with the olive oil. Loosely seal the garlic in the foil. Put on a baking sheet and bake for 1 hour. Remove from foil and cool.

Remove the garlic skin and place all ingredients in a blender. Purée until creamy.

Add more salt, pepper, tahini, or lemon juice to taste.

Serve with gluten-free pita bread, crackers, or crudités.

Free of
casein, corn, dairy, eggs, fish, gluten, nuts

Prep time
10 minutes

Total time
10 minutes

Makes
3 cups (142 1-teaspoon servings)

Per Serving
Calories: 35
Calories from fat: 6
Total fat: less than 1 g
Saturated fat: 0 g
Cholesterol: 0 mg
Sodium: 37 mg
Carbohydrates: 3 g
Fiber: 2 g
Sugars: 0 g
Protein: 5 g
Vitamin A: 2% DV
Vitamin C: 25% DV
Calcium: 2% DV
Iron: 7% DV

Variations

Use as a spread on sandwiches with sprouts, lettuce, tomato, or any other fresh vegetables.

For a lighter flavor, add fresh parsley to the blended purée.

Mexican Fiesta Rice 'n' Beans with Veggies

After eliminating gluten from my diet, I found Mexican and Spanish cuisines to be safe because they are mostly based on corn rather than wheat. If you do not have a corn allergy, you can go the same way. This dish has a wonderfully mild, spicy flavor, but is still safe and gentle for your special digestive tract.

1 cup uncooked brown rice

1 red or green bell pepper, cut into match sticks

1 large onion, diced

1 cup baby carrots, cut into match sticks

2 tablespoons olive oil

1 14.5-ounce can pinto or adzuki beans, drained

1 bunch leafy greens, such as romaine, Swiss chard, or kale, torn or chopped

1 1¼-ounce packet taco seasoning

½ cup water

1 avocado, peeled, stone removed, and diced

Blue corn chips, crushed (optional)

Free of
casein, corn, dairy, eggs, fish, gluten, nuts

Prep time
15 minutes

Total time
1 hour

Makes
4 servings

Per Serving (Without Corn Chips)
Calories: 410
Calories from fat: 115
Total fat: 13 g
Saturated fat: 2 g
Cholesterol: 0 mg
Sodium: 300 mg
Carbohydrates: 68 g
Fiber: 7 g
Sugars: 6 g
Protein: 7 g
Vitamin A: 172% DV
Vitamin C: 170% DV
Calcium: 9% DV
Iron: 12% DV

Cook the brown rice according to package directions.

While the rice is cooking, heat skillet over medium-high heat and sauté the onions, pepper, and carrot in the olive oil for 5 minutes.

Add beans and leafy greens and mix to combine. Allow greens to wilt slightly, about 2 minutes.

Add seasoning packet and water and stir to combine. Allow sauce to thicken, about 5 minutes more.

Serve the vegetable and bean mixture over brown rice. Top with avocado and corn chips.

When choosing meats, pick organic, grass-fed beef or poultry. Conventional meat is laden with pesticides, growth hormones, steroids, and antibiotics, and the cows are fed a grain-based diet consisting of corn feed that is not typical of the animal's diet. This decreases the nutritious omega-3 fatty acid content of the beef.

Simple Grilled Chicken

An excellent and easy recipe for nights when cooking is the last thing you want to do. Pair with a simple salad and you are all set. This dish is mildly anti-inflammatory.

1 pound boneless chicken breasts
2 cups barbecue sauce
2 tablespoons olive oil
½ small red onion, diced
⅓ pint cherry tomatoes, halved

Combine chicken and barbecue sauce in a shallow pan.

Heat a grill pan over an outdoor grill set at medium-high heat. Heat the olive oil in the pan. Grill the chicken for 5 minutes on each side.

Serve over brown rice and top with red onion and cherry tomatoes.

Free of
casein, corn, dairy, eggs, fish, gluten

Prep time
10 minutes

Total time
25 minutes

Makes
4 servings

Per Serving
Calories: 414
Calories from fat: 242
Total fat: 27 g
Saturated fat: 5 g
Cholesterol: 49 mg
Sodium: 575 mg
Carbohydrates: 26 g
Fiber: 2 g
Sugar: 4 g
Protein: 18 g
Vitamin A: 6% DV
Vitamin C: 10% DV
Calcium: 3% DV
Iron: 8% DV

Grilled Chicken and Shiitake Mushrooms with Polenta

This dish is strongly anti-inflammatory.

2 tablespoons olive oil

1 pound boneless chicken tenderloins

1 cup chopped shiitake mushrooms, stems removed

½ cup balsamic vinegar

½ teaspoon garlic powder

½ teaspoon onion powder

Salt and pepper to taste

1 roll of premade polenta

1 roasted red pepper, chopped (optional)

Free of
casein, dairy, eggs, fish, gluten

Prep time
5 minutes

Total time
20 minutes

Makes
4 servings

Per Serving
Calories: 547
Calories from fat: 249
Total fat: 28 g
Saturated fat: 5 g
Cholesterol: 49 mg
Sodium: 532 mg
Carbohydrates: 53 g
Fiber: 5 g
Sugar: 6 g
Protein: 21 g
Vitamin A: 7% DV
Vitamin C: 21% DV
Calcium: 4% DV
Iron: 16% DV

Prepare polenta as per package instructions.

Put the olive oil in a grill pan of an outdoor grill over high heat. Put the chicken and mushrooms in the hot pan at the same time. Grill the chicken for 3–5 minutes on each side, depending on the thickness, or until browned and no longer pink in the middle. Turn the mushrooms frequently so they do not burn.

In a small bowl, combine balsamic vinegar, garlic powder, onion powder, and salt and pepper to taste. Pour the mixture over the chicken and mushrooms and allow it to glaze for about 2 minutes. Serve the chicken and mushrooms over the polenta and top with roasted red pepper.

Chicken and Veggie Tacos

I love these homemade tacos. They are a healthy, fast option for those days when I need a break in the kitchen and still want to keep everyone pleased with my dinner choice.

6 corn taco shells

2 tablespoons olive oil

1 large onion, diced

1 cup baby carrots, cut into match sticks

½ red bell pepper, cut into match sticks

½ green bell pepper, cut into match sticks

1 pound cooked chicken, chopped, or 1 15-ounce can of black, kidney, or cannellini beans, drained

1½–2 teaspoons chili powder

1 teaspoon salt

Toppings:

1 avocado, peeled and stone removed, mashed

Shredded baby spinach

Soy cheese

Scallions

Commercial pico de gallo

Free of
citrus, dairy, eggs, fish, garlic, nuts, and mustard

Prep time
10 minutes

Total time
25 minutes

Makes
6 tacos

Per Taco
(Without Toppings)
Calories: 298
Calories from fat: 18
Total fat: 2 g
Saturated fat: 2 g
Cholesterol: 0 mg
Sodium: 252 mg
Carbohydrates: 38 g
Fiber: 7 g
Sugar: 4 g
Protein: 7 g
Vitamin A: 45% DV
Vitamin C: 72% DV
Calcium: 6% DV
Iron: 12% DV

Warm taco shells in oven according to package directions.

Heat the olive oil in a large skillet on medium heat and add the vegetables and chicken or beans, chili powder, and salt and pepper to taste. Cook for about 8–10 minutes or until veggies are slightly soft and the onion is opaque.

Put the chicken or bean mixture into the taco shells and top with your choice of condiments.

Apple Rosemary Cornish Game Hens

This recipe, courtesy of the Institute for Integrative Nutrition, was the star of a recent dinner party we threw. It is a tasty alternative to the traditional turkey, and makes more sense when you're not hosting a big crowd.

1 Cornish game hen
3 gala apples, peeled, cored, and diced
1 cup fresh or thawed cranberries
½ cup apple juice or cider
½ cup maple syrup
4 sprigs fresh rosemary
2 teaspoons curry powder
Salt and freshly cracked pepper to taste

Free of
casein, corn, dairy, eggs, fish, gluten

Prep time
10 minutes

Total time
1 hour

Makes
2 servings

Per Serving
Calories: 387
Calories from fat: 112
Total fat: 12 g
Saturated fat: 3 g
Cholesterol: 84 mg
Sodium: 50 mg
Carbohydrates: 56 g
Fiber: 4 g
Sugar: 46 g
Protein: 15 g
Vitamin A: 3% DV
Vitamin C: 48% DV
Calcium: 6% DV
Iron: 10% DV

Preheat oven to 400°F.

Remove the giblets from the Cornish hen, rinse, and pat dry. Save the giblets for another use. Slice the hens in half, starting at the top of the breastbone. Sprinkle with salt and pepper. Line a large, shallow baking dish with aluminum foil and set the hen halves side by side with the skin side up. Tuck a rosemary sprig under each half.

To make the sauce, combine the apples, cranberries, maple syrup, apple juice, curry, and the remaining rosemary sprigs in a saucepan over medium-high heat. Bring to a boil, stirring frequently. Decrease the heat to low, cover, and simmer, stirring frequently, until the apple pieces are very soft and the berries have broken open and released their juices. This will take about 8–10 minutes.

Brush the sauce on the hens to coat, and bake for 25 minutes, or until they reach an internal temperature of 180°F. While baking, baste once or twice with the sauce, reserving the rest.

Remove the hens from the roasting pan and keep warm. Pour the juices from the pan into the remaining sauce and bring to a boil. Reduce to simmer until the sauce thickens, about 3 minutes.

Serve the hens with the sauce on the side.

Orange Marmalade Turkey Burgers

I developed this recipe when I was looking for a way to keep turkey burgers moist and I decided to try some leftover marmalade I had on hand. Now I make it a point to always have it around. If you don't have orange marmalade, apricot jam or cranberry sauce will work just as well.

1 pound ground turkey
½ red bell pepper, chopped
3 scallions, both the white and green parts, sliced
2 heaping tablespoons orange marmalade
1 tablespoon poultry seasoning
½ teaspoon salt
Pinch red pepper flake
2 tablespoons olive oil

Combine the first seven ingredients in a large bowl and mix well. Divide into four equal portions and form into patties.

Place a grill pan on an outdoor grill over high heat. Heat the olive oil in the pan and grill the burgers for 3–5 minutes on each side, or until golden and cooked through.

Free of
casein, corn, dairy, eggs, fish, gluten

Prep time
10 minutes

Total time
20 minutes

Makes
4 servings

Per Serving
Calories: 317
Calories from fat: 157
Total fat: 17 g
Saturated fat: 4 g
Cholesterol: 134 mg
Sodium: 168 mg
Carbohydrates: 9 g
Fiber: 1 g
Sugar: 7 g
Protein: 30 g
Vitamin A: 14% DV
Vitamin C: 44% DV
Calcium: 4% DV
Iron: 13% DV

Curry Turkey Tenders

This main meal tastes salty, smoky, and sweet. The smokiness from the curry is balanced nicely by the tartness from the apple cider. The coconut oil adds an element of surprise that will have guests wondering about the mysterious flavor.

2 tablespoons coconut oil
4 4-ounce turkey cutlets
1 apple, peeled, cored, and sliced
⅔ cup apple juice or cider
1 tablespoon curry powder
Freshly ground pepper to taste

Heat the oil in a large skillet over medium-high heat. Add the turkey cutlets in one layer and place the apple slices in between them. Sauté the cutlets for 5–8 minutes on each side until brown.

Pour in apple juice and add the curry powder and ground pepper. Reduce the heat to low, cover, and simmer until cooked through, about 10 minutes.

Free of
casein, corn, dairy, eggs, fish, gluten

Prep time
5 minutes

Total time
25 minutes

Makes
2 servings

Per Serving
Calories: 98
Calories from fat: 34
Total fat: 4 g
Saturated fat: 3 g
Cholesterol: 18 mg
Sodium: 14 mg
Carbohydrates: 9 g
Fiber: 1 g
Sugar: 7 g
Protein: 7 g
Vitamin A: 1% DV
Vitamin C: 27% DV
Iron: 5% DV
Calcium: 1% DV

Mom's Mind-Blowing Stir-Fry

As a child, egg noodles were one of my most requested side dishes. Now on my "no-no" list, I was in search of a tasty new type of noodle to satisfy my cravings. Voilà! One day, I was browsing through the Asian foods aisle while shopping with my mother, and I discovered a gluten-free must have: rice noodles. Mom and I decided to try them out in a stir-fry and found a winner.

1 16-ounce package Asian rice noodles

1 teaspoon olive oil

2½ pounds chicken tenders, cut into 1-inch slices

3 tablespoons gluten-free tamari

2 tablespoons sesame oil

2 1-pound packages frozen stir-fry vegetables

Sesame seeds for garnish

Salt and pepper to taste

Prepare rice noodles according to package directions. Drain and set aside.

Free of
casein, corn, dairy, eggs, fish, gluten

Prep time
10 minutes

Total time
25 minutes

Makes
4 servings

Per Serving
Calories: 361
Calories from fat: 179
Total fat: 20 g
Saturated fat: 4 g
Cholesterol: 33 mg
Sodium: 859 mg
Carbohydrates: 31 g
Fiber: 3 g
Sugar: 1 g
Protein: 15 g
Vitamin A: 15% DV
Vitamin C: 45% DV
Calcium: 7% DV
Iron: 11% DV

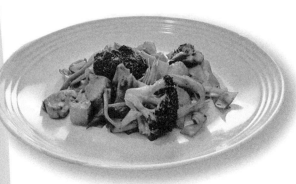

Heat the olive oil in a large skillet or wok over high heat. Add the chicken to the hot oil and stir. Add ½ of the tamari and ½ of the sesame oil.

Stir-fry for 5 minutes, or until vegetables and chicken are completely cooked through.

Add frozen vegetables and stir-fry for about 3 more minutes, or until incorporated. Add remaining tamari and sesame oil.

Reduce the heat, cover, and cook for 5 more minutes. Add the noodles to stir-fry and cook for 3 minutes. Add more tamari and sesame oil, if desired. Sprinkle with sesame seeds and add salt and pepper to taste. Serve immediately.

Oven-Roasted Chicken and Potatoes

This recipe was inspired by my friend Phil, who was awesome at lending me recipe advice for this book. His input and insight was greatly appreciated and paid off, as you will see. Round out the meal with steamed broccoli.

1 whole chicken, about 4 pounds

3 tablespoons olive oil

¼ cup chopped fresh oregano

Juice of 2 lemons

Salt and pepper

4 cups free-range chicken stock

4 sweet potatoes, cut in to ½-inch chunks, skins left on

Free of
casein, corn, dairy, eggs, fish, gluten

Prep time
10 minutes

Total time
2 hours

Makes
6 servings

Per Serving
Calories: 388
Calories from fat: 183
Total fat: 20 g
Saturated fat: 5 g
Cholesterol: 88 mg
Sodium: 497 mg
Carbohydrates: 22 g
Fiber: 3 g
Sugar: 5 g
Protein: 29 g
Vitamin A: 262% DV
Vitamin C: 16% DV
Calcium: 5% DV
Iron: 12% DV

Preheat oven to 350°F.

Remove the giblets from the chicken, wash and pat dry. Save the giblets for another use. Put the chicken in a deep baking pan lined with aluminum foil (no rack is necessary).

Combine the olive oil, oregano, lemon juice, and salt and pepper to taste and then rub the mixture into the flesh of the chicken. Arrange the sweet potatoes around the bird. Pour chicken broth over the potatoes, but not the chicken.

Cover tentlike with aluminum foil and bake for 1 hour. Remove foil and bake for an additional 45 minutes. Let the chicken sit for about 20 minutes before slicing.

Slow Cook Beef Tender

This fall-off-the-bone, slow-cooked beef is perfect for a cold winter Sunday dinner. And it will help you regain strength after a flare-up, as the meat is a highly absorbable source of protein. Serve it over brown rice with a side of steamed broccoli or butternut squash.

2 tablespoons olive oil
2 pounds beef short ribs, cut into pieces
1 cup warm water, more as needed
1 large Vidalia onion, chopped
2 garlic cloves, chopped
2 carrots, chopped
3 teaspoons sesame oil
5 teaspoons gluten-free tamari
5 teaspoons honey
2 scallions, chopped

Free of
casein, corn, dairy, eggs, fish, gluten

Prep time
15 minutes

Total time
About 2½ hours

Makes
4 servings

Per Serving
Calories: 295
Calories from fat: 166
Total fat: 19 g
Saturated fat: 5 g
Cholesterol: 38 mg
Sodium: 868 mg
Carbohydrates: 19 g
Fiber: 1 g
Sugar: 6 g
Protein: 14 g
Vitamin A: 15% DV
Vitamin C: 5% DV
Calcium: 2% DV
Iron: 11% DV

Heat the olive oil in a large stockpot over medium-high heat. When hot, add the beef. Cook, turning until browned, about 10 minutes. Reduce heat to low and add water; take care while doing this as the oil may splatter. Cover.

Cook the meat so it continues browning, stirring occasional. As the water evaporates, add more as needed so the beef does not burn. You must keep up this process over the next hour and a half. Stay close to the stove and check in on the dish every 10 minutes or so in case you need to add more water.

Add the onions, garlic, carrots, sesame oil, tamari, and honey and cook for another half hour. Add the pepper and serve garnished with the scallions.

Simply Classic Lemon Pepper Rosemary Chicken

Get your lemon on and protect your immune system! Lemon is great because of its high vitamin C content. This recipe pairs very well with Lemon Basil Quinoa (see recipe on page 212).

4 ¼-pound boneless chicken breasts

Pinch coarsely ground black pepper

4–5 fresh rosemary sprigs, spikes removed and chopped

Zest and juice of 2 lemons

4 tablespoons olive oil

Salt and pepper to taste

Coat chicken on both sides with black pepper. Season lightly with salt. Set aside.

Combine the rosemary with the olive oil and the lemon zest and juice. Heat a large skillet over medium-high heat. Add marinade.

Add the chicken breasts to the marinade and sauté for 6–7 minutes on each side, until cooked through, basting with marinade as needed to keep the chicken lightly covered while it cooks. Transfer to a serving platter and brush with the remaining marinade.

Free of
casein, corn, dairy, eggs, fish, gluten

Prep time
10 minutes

Total time
25 minutes

Makes
4 servings

Per Serving
Calories: 455
Calories from fat: 299
Total fat: 33 g
Saturated fat: 6 g
Cholesterol: 49 mg
Sodium: 513 mg
Carbohydrates: 23 g
Fiber: 2 g
Sugar: 1 g
Protein: 18 g
Vitamin A: 1% DV
Vitamin C: 19% DV
Calcium: 3% DV
Iron: 8% DV

Certain fish, such as sardines, mackerel, tuna, and salmon are high in omega-3 fatty acids, which are known to help reduce inflammation. They have been playing a big part in IBD-friendly diets since the late 1970s.

These recipes are chock-full of the healthy fish listed above, which are available for purchase at most grocery stores. Whenever possible, choose wild fish rather than those that have been farm raised, as wild ones contain less mercury and are richer in flavor.

Grilled Halibut Steaks with Mustard

For me, there is nothing like a fresh, wild-caught halibut steak in the summer. The mustard seasoning makes this simply delicious. Pair it with grilled zucchini and peppers for a light dinner.

4 7-ounce halibut steaks
1 teaspoon ground cumin
2 tablespoon brown mustard
Salt and pepper to taste
1 tablespoon olive oil
1 lemon, cut into wedges

Sprinkle the halibut with cumin, salt, and pepper. Spread mustard over the fish on both sides.

Heat grill pan over an outdoor grill to medium high heat. Heat the olive oil in the pan and grill the fish for 5 minutes on each side, or until cooked through. Serve with lemon wedges.

Free of
casein, corn, dairy, eggs, gluten, nuts

Prep time
10 minutes

Cook time
20 minutes

Makes
4 servings

Per Serving
Calories: 264
Calories from fat: 74
Total fat: 8 g
Saturated fat: 1 g
Cholesterol: 64 mg
Sodium: 141 mg
Carbohydrates: 2 g
Fiber: 0 g
Sugars: 0 g
Protein: 43 g
Vitamin A: 7% DV
Vitamin C: 9% DV
Calcium: 11% DV
Iron: 15% DV

Grilled Salmon with Honey Ginger Sauce

Serve this grilled fish with roasted broccoli and a baked sweet potato sprinkled with cinnamon. This recipe utilizes a grill pan, which serves as a wonderful alternative to an outdoor grill. A grill pan is a deep fry pan with grooves on the bottom. Grill pans can be purchased from stores like Target or Wal-Mart.

3 tablespoons orange marmalade

1 teaspoon honey

1 teaspoon grated fresh ginger

Juice of 2 limes

1 pinch salt and pepper

2 salmon steaks, about 4 ounces each

3 tablespoons olive oil

Preheat an indoor grill pan to high. Combine the marmalade, honey, ginger, lime juice, and salt and pepper in a small mixing bowl.

Heat the oil in a grill pan. Grill the steaks in the oil for 5 minutes on each side. Generously brush the fish with the marinade several times while cooking.

Free of
casein, corn, dairy, eggs, gluten, nuts

Prep time
10 minutes

Total time
20 minutes

Makes
4 servings

Per Serving
Calories: 360
Calories from fat: 150
Total fat: 15 g
Saturated fat: 3 g
Cholesterol: 109 mg
Sodium: 120 mg
Carbohydrates: 0 g
Fiber: 0 g
Sugars: 2 g
Protein: 40 g
Vitamin A: 6% DV
Vitamin C: 14% DV
Calcium: 4% DV
Iron: 11% DV

Baked Coconut Shrimp

This is a simple and delicous variation of the original heavy, fried version. This is always a hit at parties or as an appetizer. It is also excellent for dinner, served with brown rice with peas and a salad.

2 dozen jumbo shrimp, shells removed and deveined

1 15-ounce can coconut milk

1 cup cornstarch or rice flour

1 12-ounce package unsweetened coconut flakes

Coconut oil for baking

¼ cup orange marmalade, for dipping

Preheat oven to 375°F.

Grease large cookie or baking sheet with coconut oil.

Pour coconut milk into a large mixing bowl. Pour corn starch or rice flour onto a large plate, sheet, or parchment paper. Spread the coconut flakes on another plate.

Dip each shrimp into cornstarch, then into coconut milk, and then roll in coconut flakes. Place on baking sheet. Repeat the process until completed. Bake until golden brown, about 15–20 minutes.

Serve with orange marmalade or eat plain.

Free of
casein, dairy, eggs, gluten, nuts

Prep time
15 minutes

Total time
30 minutes

Makes
4 servings

Per Serving (With Dipping Sauce)
Calories: 312
Calories from fat: 89
Total fat: 10g
Saturated fat: 8 g
Cholesterol: 46 mg
Sodium: 116 mg
Carbohydrates: 45g
Fiber: 4 g
Sugar: 10g
Protein: 10g
Vitamin A. 6% DV
Vitamin C: 1% DV
Calcium: 7%
Iron: 11%

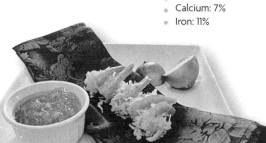

Our Favorite Salmon

I used to despise salmon, but that changed a few years ago while I was vacationing at Disney World. On a whim, I decided to try salmon at a character dinner with Winnie the Pooh and Tigger. I was amazed at how much I loved it. I asked the chef for the recipe, and he e-mailed it to me! This is my version of my favorite "Disney" salmon, using my easy organic store-bought pesto and swapping out unhealthy sugars for maple syrup. If you don't like the heat of peppers, you can substitute roasted bell peppers.

4 wild salmon fillets, about 7 ounces each
2 dried ancho chilies
1 cup water
2 tablespoons olive oil
¼ cup pure maple syrup
Salt and pepper
1 cup commercial pesto

Free of
casein, corn, eggs, gluten, nuts

Prep time
20 minutes

Total time
2½ hours

Makes
4 servings

Per Serving
Calories: 438
Calories from fat: 208
Total fat: 23 g
Saturated fat: 4 g
Cholesterol: 109 mg
Sodium: 187 mg
Carbohydrates: 16 g
Fiber: 1 g
Sugars: 12 g
Protein: 40 g
Vitamin A: 24% DV
Vitamin C: 4% DV
Calcium: 5% DV
Iron: 13% DV

Preheat the oven to 375°F.

Put the dried chilies and the water in a medium sauce pan. Bring to a simmer and cook for about 10 minutes or until chilies are reconstituted and soft.

Wearing disposable plastic or rubber gloves, remove the stems and seeds from the chilies, and discard. Chop the chilies; add them along with olive oil, maple syrup, and salt and pepper to a food processor; and blend until a smooth paste forms.

Arrange the salmon in a baking dish and cover with the paste. Marinate it for at least 1 hour in the refrigerator, flipping it once or twice. Alternatively, you can marinate it overnight.

Remove the fish and bring to room temperature.
Bake for 15 minutes. Another option would be to grill the fish. Serve with pesto sauce drizzled over the top.

Sesame Glazed Ginger Tuna Steaks with Brown Rice

One day I was really craving Rice-A-Roni, which I used to love. However, these days I like to control the ingredients in my food, so I came up with my own version. Recently, I teamed it up with tuna and, Wow, I liked what I got! Steamed carrots with honey and ginger complement this dish well.

1 cup uncooked brown rice
1 pound tuna steaks
1 cup of sesame ginger stir-fry sauce
3 tablespoons sesame oil
4 medium carrots, cut into match sticks
1 cup halved snow peas
2 scallions, chopped on an angle

Marinate the tuna in ginger sauce for at least 30 minutes. While the tuna is marinating, cook the brown rice according to the package instructions.

Preheat the grill pan to medium high heat. Add sesame oil to pan, along with tuna steaks. Grill the fish for 3–4 minutes on each side, until no longer pink. If you would like a rawer, more-pink fish, grill for only 2 minutes per side. Transfer to a plate and keep warm.

Heat the sesame oil in a grill pan. Stir-fry the carrots and snow peas for 3–4 minutes. Add cooked brown rice and heat through, about 4 minutes, stirring constantly.

Serve tuna on top of rice. Add scallions on top.

Free of
casein, corn, dairy, eggs, gluten, nuts

Prep time
15 minutes

Total time
1 hour

Makes
4 servings

Per Serving
Calories: 316
Calories from fat: 106
Total fat: 12 g
Saturated fat: 2 g
Cholesterol: 32 mg
Sodium: 157 mg
Carbohydrates: 25 g
Fiber: 6 g
Sugars: 3 g
Protein: 25 g
Vitamin A: 121% DV
Vitamin C: 4% DV
Calcium: 3% DV
Iron: 12% DV

Grains can be a welcome part of your diet when you have IBD, so I encourage you to enjoy them. Stick to the gluten-free grains featured here to avoid having any type of difficulty with digestion. The following recipes feature easy-to-breakdown whole grains that contain a lot of B-complex vitamins, which help you sustain high energy levels for prolonged periods of time.

Tomato and Pasta Salad

Pasta and tomatoes are a perfect pair. This simple, healthy salad makes a nice lunch alongside a homemade vegetable soup.

1 8-ounce box penne brown rice pasta, cooked and cooled

1 pint cherry tomatoes, whole or halved lengthwise

5 tablespoons extra virgin olive oil

2 garlic cloves, minced

Salt and pepper to taste

2 tablespoons balsamic vinegar

2 sundried tomatoes packed in olive oil

1 cup tightly packed arugula

Combine the olive oil and garlic, with salt and pepper to taste in a small bowl.

Put the pasta, tomatoes, and arugula in a large bowl. Whisk the dressing and pour over the pasta. Combine well and serve.

Free of
gluten, dairy, eggs, soy, corn, fish, nuts

Prep time
10 minutes

Total time
20 minutes

Makes
6 servings

Per Serving
Calories: 146
Calories from fat: 98
Total Fat: 11 g
Saturated Fat: 1 g
Cholesterol: 0 mg
Sodium: 140 mg
Carbohydrates: 27 g
Fiber: 2 g
Sugars: 4 g
Protein: 3 g
Vitamin A: 8% DV
Vitamin C: 19% DV
Calcium: 3% DV
Iron: 5% DV

Authentic and Easy Fried Rice

I love fried rice, but I like to make my own healthy version. This recipe substitutes brown rice for the traditional white rice used in most Chinese restaurants. This dish also avoids MSG, without sacrificing flavor. It is quite filling, so I like to have it as a shared main entrée. You can also serve it as a side dish with some broccoli and baked chicken.

2–3 tablespoons sesame oil
2 tablespoons gluten-free tamari
1 small onion, diced
1 clove garlic, chopped
2 cups leftover brown rice
2 scallions, chopped on an angle
1 egg (optional)
Pinch crushed red pepper flake (optional)

Heat the oil in a large skillet over medium high heat and add the tamari, onion, and garlic. Sauté for about 5 minutes or until the onions are translucent. Stir in the rice and heat through, about 5 minutes.

Add scallions and egg (if using). Keep stirring the rice to incorporate the egg. Add crushed red pepper flakes, if using.

Free of
casein, corn, dairy, eggs, fish, gluten, nuts

Prep time
10 minutes

Total time
20 minutes

Makes
4 servings

Per Serving
Calories: 443
Calories from fat: 93
Total fat: 11 g
Saturated fat: 2 g
Cholesterol: 53 mg
Sodium: 545 mg
Carbohydrates: 77 g
Fiber: 4 g
Sugars: 2 g
Protein: 10 g
Vitamin A: 1% DV
Vitamin C: 5% DV
Calcium: 5% DV
Iron: 12%

Little Lunch Box Mini Pizzas

The love of pizza is universal. These mini pies are perfect for kids and adults alike and they don't contain dairy or gluten. Vegan Parma is an excellent dairy-free cheese substitute made from walnuts. As it turns out, toasted walnuts and salt taste surprisingly similar to actual Parmesan cheese.

2 small allergen-free whole-grain French rolls (they are about the size of an English muffin)
1 cup commercial tomato sauce
½ cup vegan Parmesan cheese substitute (I recommend Vegan Parma Cheese Substitute)

Any topping or combination of toppings of your choice:
Sautéed onions
Bell peppers
Raw broccoli florets
Pineapple pieces
Pepperoni

Preheat oven to 350°F.

Slice the rolls in half and place on a large cookie sheet, cut side up. Spread the slices with tomato sauce.

Top the tomato sauce with vegan Parmesan cheese substitute. Add additional toppings of choice.

Bake for 10 minutes.

Free of
casein, corn, dairy, eggs, fish, gluten

Prep time
5 minutes

Total time
15 minutes

Makes
4 mini pizzas

Per Pizza (Without Additional Toppings)
Calories: 322
Calories from fat: 178
Total fat: 21 g
Saturated fat: 2 g
Cholesterol: 0 mg
Sodium: 229 mg
Carbohydrates: 29 g
Fiber: 4 g
Sugars: 5 g
Protein: 8 g
Vitamin A: 10% DV
Vitamin C: 14% DV
Calcium: 7% DV
Iron: 13% DV

Cashew Rice Noodles

Many people enjoy noodles with peanut sauce, but I got nutty and decided to replace the peanuts with cashews, my favorite nut. I then kicked things up a notch and made the sauce gluten free by using rice noodles instead of the traditional wheat-flour ones.

½ 8-ounce package rice noodles
1 cup shredded radicchio
½ red bell pepper, chopped into match sticks
½ cup shredded carrots
½ cup roasted and salted cashews
1 bunch scallions, both white and green parts, chopped

For the cashew butter sauce:
½ cup cashew butter
2 cloves garlic, minced
¼ cup orange juice
4 teaspoons gluten-free tamari

Free of
casein, corn, dairy, eggs, fish, gluten

Prep time
5 minutes

Total time
15 minutes

Makes
6 servings

Per Serving
Calories: 395
Calories from fat: 202
Total fat: 24 g
Saturated fat: 5 g
Cholesterol: 0 mg
Sodium: 1,035 mg
Carbohydrates: 37 g
Fiber: 3 g
Sugars: 8 g
Protein: 12 g
Vitamin A: 52% DV
Vitamin C: 141% DV
Calcium: 6% DV
Iron: 21% DV

Fill a large pot halfway with water. Boil, then turn off the heat and soak the rice noodles for 10 minutes. Drain, rinse, and cool.

While the noodles are soaking, make the cashew butter sauce. Mix all the ingredients in a bowl, whisking with a fork to blend. Add a little water to thin it to the consistency of a sauce.

Put the noodles in a large bowl and add the radicchio, red pepper, and carrots. Add the sauce, and toss well to combine. Garnish with the cashews and scallions and then serve.

Lemon and Basil Quinoa

The hallmark of this wonderful grain is the vitality you'll feel after eating it. Here it is made into a citrusy, light salad. In addition to great flavor, you'll get nutritious B-complex vitamins and amino acids.

2½ cups vegetable broth

1½ cups dry roasted quinoa

Zest of 2 lemons

½ cup chopped toasted walnuts

2 tablespoons chopped fresh basil

1 tablespoon olive oil

3 tablespoons dried cranberries (optional)

Bring the vegetable broth to a simmer in a medium saucepan and stir in the quinoa. Bring back to a low boil, cover, and cook over low heat for 12 minutes. Remove from heat and let stand for 5 minutes.

Fluff with a fork and toss in lemon, basil, and toasted walnuts. Add cranberries, if desired. Allow salad to chill in the refrigerator for 2 hours.

Free of
casein, corn, dairy, eggs, fish, gluten

Prep time
5 minutes

Total time
20 minutes plus 2 hours, unattended

Makes
4 servings

Per Serving
Calories: 390
Calories from fat: 210
Total fat: 24 g
Saturated fat: 3 g
Cholesterol: 0 mg
Sodium: 95 mg
Carbohydrates: 37 g
Fiber: 5 g
Sugars: 6 g
Protein: 9 g
Vitamin A: 3% DV
Vitamin C: 13% DV
Calcium: 4% DV
Iron: 15% DV

Almond Millet Pilaf

I make this for my son on winter mornings to get us up and going. This pilaf is simple, and can be made as a side dish, breakfast, or even dessert, depending on how you modify the flavors. For a sweeter breakfast or dessert, you can add maple syrup and cinnamon. For a dinner side dish, cook as directed below.

3 cups water
1 cup millet
1 teaspoon salt
1 teaspoon almond extract
1 tablespoon minced fresh ginger
¼ cup toasted almonds (optional)

Bring the water to a boil. While the water is boiling, rinse the millet in a strainer to remove any dirt and bitterness. Add millet to water. Reduce the heat and simmer 20 minutes. Drain.

Transfer millet to medium mixing bowl and add salt, extract, almonds, and ginger. Stir.

Free of
casein, corn, dairy, eggs, fish, gluten

Prep time
5 minutes

Total time
30 minutes

Makes
4 servings

Per Serving
Calories: 160
Calories from fat: 15
Total fat: 2 g
Saturated fat: 0 g
Cholesterol: 0 mg
Sodium: 5 mg
Carbohydrates: 30 g
Sugars: 0 g
Protein: 5 g
Vitamin A: 0%DV
Vitamin C: 0% DV
Calcium: 3% DV
Iron: 6% DV

Roasted Cauliflower and White Wine Pasta

I enjoy cauliflower sauce as a pleasant change from traditional tomato sauce. This sauce provides a rich, creamy taste that has you thinking you are eating something really bad for you when you are not! It's a staple dish in our home, and I hope it will be in yours, too.

1 head garlic
1 head cauliflower, florets only, chopped
2 tablespoons olive oil
1 8-ounce box brown rice pasta
½ cup white wine
16 basil leaves, torn or shredded
Salt and pepper to taste

Free of
casein, corn, dairy, eggs, fish, gluten

Prep time
10 minutes

Total time
1½ hours

Makes
4 servings

Per Serving
Calories: 265
Calories from fat: 69
Total fat: 8 g
Cholesterol: 0 mg
Sodium: 70 mg
Carbohydrates: 37 g
Sugar: 5 g
Protein: 7 g
Vitamin A: 3% DV
Vitamin C: 168% DV
Calcium: 8% DV
Iron: 9% DV

Preheat oven to 500°F or broil.

Remove the stem from the garlic, while keeping the skin intact. Wrap the head in aluminum foil and roast for 1 hour. Remove garlic and, when cool enough to handle, remove the skin.

Reduce oven to 350°F.

Arrange the cauliflower in a shallow glass baking dish and coat with the olive oil. Bake for 30 minutes.

Meanwhile, bring a large pot of water to a boil and cook pasta according to package directions.

Put the roasted cauliflower and garlic in a large skillet and then add the pasta, white wine, and basil. Cook for 2–3 minutes over medium-high heat to evaporate the alcohol. Add salt and pepper to taste.

Rice Noodles in Basil Butter Sauce

Yum—basil and noodles! What a wonderful culinary marriage. Organic basil has a sweet, earthy flavor that gets the taste buds going every time.

1-pound package uncooked rice noodles
1 cup coarsely chopped walnuts
3 tablespoons butter substitute (I recommend Earth Balance [www.earthbalance.com] and Smart Balance organic butter substitutes. They are dairy free and soy free.)
½ cup chicken or vegetable broth
16 leaves basil, torn or chopped
1 clove garlic, chopped
1 large Portobello mushroom, diced
Salt and pepper to taste

Cook the rice noodles according to package directions. Drain and set aside.

While the pasta is cooking, heat the walnuts in a small heavy-bottom dry skillet, tossing and stirring to toast, about 4 minutes.

Melt the butter in a large skillet. Add the garlic and sauté for 2 minutes. Do not let it burn. Add the chicken broth and stir to incorporate. Add mushroom, cook 3 minutes more. Add basil and salt and pepper.

Toss noodles with basil butter sauce and toasted walnuts and serve.

Free of
casein, corn, dairy, eggs, fish, gluten

Prep time
10 minutes

Total time
30 minutes

Makes
4 servings

Per Serving
Calories: 378
Calories from fat: 230
Total fat: 27 g
Saturated fat: 4 g
Cholesterol: 1 mg
Sodium: 141 mg
Carbohydrates: 29 g
Fiber: 4 g
Sugar: 1 g
Protein: 8 g
Vitamin A: 14% DV
Vitamin C: 1% DV
Calcium: 4% DV
Iron: 8% DV

VEGETABLES

People with IBD are often told that they should be wary of vegetables, as they are packed with fiber and can be a bit difficult to break down. This is true, but as long as you cook your vegetables properly and ensure to you are getting your daily intake of whole grains in your diet, it is unlikely you will have any issues with the digestion at all!

Interestingly enough, it is protein, not vegetables, that I find to be the culprit when I do food-sensitivities testing on clients. Try adding vegetables back into your diet slowly and see how you feel. You may be surprised to find that you can tolerate them well!

We all know we should eat lots of green vegetables—at least one serving a day. Dark, green leafy vegetables are extra important if you have IBD. Studies show that greens help promote healthy intestinal flora, which refers to the beneficial bacteria that help support your immune system. For those with IBD this is crucial to maintaining your health and can prevent infections, clear out mucus, strengthen your immune system, and purify the liver, kidneys, and lungs!

For some people with IBD, eating raw greens aggravates the tender intestinal system. If this is the case with you, dress your greens with a sweet fruit juice, such as apple and kiwi, which will allow the greens to breakdown easier. If this isn't your cup of tea, you can always boil greens until they are soft or add them directly into soups.

The bottom line is, you need your greens. They are rich in everything you need—vitamins, minerals, and antioxidant phytonutrients.

Roasted Lemon Broccoli

This is, hands down, my favorite way to make broccoli! It's also very nutritious—it's extremely high in vitamin C and is very anti-inflammatory!

1 bunch broccoli
2 cloves garlic, minced
Juice of one lemon
2 tablespoons olive oil
Pinch of salt

Preheat oven to 350°F.

Break the broccoli into florets. Put the garlic, lemon, and olive oil in a shallow baking dish and toss to coat. Season with salt and pepper to taste. Bake for 15–20 minutes, or until lightly browned around the edges.

Free of
casein, corn, dairy, eggs, fish, gluten

Prep time
5 minutes

Total time
15 minutes

Makes
4 servings

Per Serving
Calories: 80
Calories from fat: 61
Total fat: 7 g
Saturated fat: 1 g
Cholesterol: 0 mg
Sodium: 15 mg
Carbohydrates: 4 g
Fiber: 0 g
Sugar: 0 g
Protein: 2 g
Vitamin A: 32% DV
Vitamin C: 93% DV
Calcium: 3% DV
Iron: 3% DV

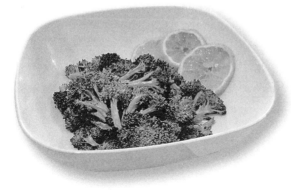

Simple Roasted Swiss Chard

Many people who come to see me have never eaten or worked with Swiss chard. Its health benefits are astounding due to its high content of antioxidant vitamins. Here is a quick recipe to acquaint you with this quite tasty leafy green. This dish is moderately anti-inflammatory.

1 bunch Swiss chard
1 clove garlic, diced
Juice of 1 lemon
Salt and pepper to taste

Preheat oven to 350°F.

Wash and chop the chard. Be sure to discard the stems, as they are hard to digest. Place the greens into a shallow glass baking dish and sprinkle with the garlic, lemon juice, and salt and pepper to taste. Bake for 15–20 minutes, or until slightly browned.

Free of
casein, corn, dairy, eggs, fish, gluten

Prep time
5 minutes

Total time
15 minutes

Makes
4 servings

Per Serving
Calories: 38
Calories from fat: 30
Total fat: 3 g
Saturated fat: 0 g
Cholesterol: 0 mg
Sodium: 39 mg
Carbohydrates: 2 g
Fiber: 0 g
Sugar: 0 g
Protein: 0 g
Vitamin A: 22% DV
Vitamin C: 19% DV
Calcium: 1% DV
Iron: 2% DV

Sweet Collard Green Stuffing

I have made this dish countless times for my local celiac support group meeting, and I always get requests for seconds. This popular Southern green is sweet, spicy, hearty, and friendly on the waistline all at the same time! Serve it with Orange Marmalade Turkey Burgers (page 196) and Comfort Cranberry Sauce (page 253). This dish is moderately anti-inflammatory.

4 tablespoons olive oil

2 ribs celery, diced

3 apples, cored and diced, skins left on

1 medium sweet onion, diced

1 carrot, grated

1 large bunch collard greens, center rib removed and coarsely chopped

3 tablespoons pumpkin pie spice

Salt and pepper to taste

Heat olive oil in a large skillet over medium high heat. Add chopped onions, carrots, celery, and apples and cook for 5–6 minutes, stirring frequently.

Add pumpkin pie spice and salt and pepper to taste. Stir in the collards and cook for 12 minutes.

Free of
casein, corn, dairy, eggs, fish, gluten

Prep time
10 minutes

Total time
25 minutes

Makes
4 servings

Per Serving (Stuffing Only)
Calories: 64
Calories from fat: 6
Total fat: less than 1 g
Saturated fat: 0 g
Cholesterol: 0 mg
Sodium: 27 mg
Carbohydrates: 15 g
Fiber: 3 g
Sugar: 8 g
Protein: 1 g
Vitamin A: 37% DV
Vitamin C: 22% DV
Calcium: 8% DV
Iron: 6% DV

Grilled Asparagus, Rice, and Peas

A simple casserole for busy evenings! I recommend using Amy's-brand soups, which you can find in the all-natural aisle in most grocery stores. This recipe is mildly anti-inflammatory.

1 14-ounce can vegan split pea soup
½ cup Enriching Eggless Mayo (see recipe on page 255)
½ teaspoon curry powder
1 bunch asparagus stalks
1 cup cooked wild rice
1 medium Vidalia onion, sliced into thin rings

Preheat oven to 375°F.

Heat grill pan to high heat, and add asparagus. Grill for 3–5 minutes, until browned. Set aside.

Combine the pea soup, mayonnaise, and curry powder in a large bowl.

Arrange the asparagus on the bottom of a shallow baking dish. Top with the wild rice. Pour the soup mixture over top of the rice. Arrange onion rings on top.

Bake the casserole for 30 minutes, or until onions looks crispy and brown.

Free of
casein, corn, dairy, eggs, fish, gluten

Prep time
15 minutes

Total time
45 minutes

Makes
8 servings

Per Serving
Calories: 183
Calories from fat: 40
Total fat: 4 g
Saturated fat: 1 g
Cholesterol: 0 mg
Sodium: 18 mg
Carbohydrates: 30 g
Fiber: 5 g
Sugar: 7 g
Protein: 7 g
Vitamin A: 6% DV
Vitamin C: 10% DV
Calcium: 4% DV
Iron: 12%

Summery Spaghetti Squash

If you have never tried spaghetti squash, check it out. I think it is wonderful and makes an excellent alternative to traditional pasta.

2 spaghetti squashes, each about 7 inches long
1 cup toasted walnuts, chopped
3 tablespoons salt
Black pepper to taste

Preheat oven to 375°F.

Slice the squash in half lengthwise and put on a baking sheet. Bake for 30–45 minutes, or until squash is soft.

When squash is baking, mix the walnuts with the salt and pepper in a small bowl. Set aside.

Remove the squash from the oven. Run the tines of a fork back and forth over the flesh until a spaghetti-like shape forms. Repeat until you are down to the squash skin. Discard skins. Transfer to a large bowl and add the walnuts.

Free of
casein, corn, dairy, eggs, fish, gluten

Prep time
5 minutes

Total time
45 minutes

Makes
4 servings

Per Serving
Calories: 223
Calories from fat: 164
Total fat: 20 g
Saturated fat: 2 g
Cholesterol: 0 mg
Sodium: 42 mg
Carbohydrates: 11 g
Fiber: 2 g
Sugar: 1 g
Protein: 5 g
Vitamin A: 1% DV
Vitamin C: 4% DV
Calcium: 5% DV
Iron: 6% DV

Roasted Carrots with Molasses and Dill

Carrots are high in beta carotene, which is wonderful for the immune system. Molasses is high in magnesium, potassium, and phosphorus. When your IBD is acting up, one of the first things you should be concerned about is replacing valuable electrolytes and minerals. This dish is chock-full of minerals, therefore perfect to eat during or after a flare-up to replenish and rebalance the body's vitamin stores. This recipe is mildly anti-inflammatory.

1 pound baby carrots

2 medium parsnips, peeled and chopped into
    2-inch pieces

2 tablespoons olive oil

2 tablespoons molasses

½ teaspoon salt

2 teaspoons fresh dill, chopped

Preheat oven to 425°F.

Arrange the carrots and parsnips in a shallow baking dish. Mix oil, molasses, and salt, and pour over the top.

Cover and bake for 30 minutes. Uncover and bake for 15 more minutes. Sprinkle fresh dill over the top. Serve warm.

Free of
casein, corn, dairy, eggs, fish, gluten

Prep time
5 minutes

Total time
50 minutes

Makes
4 servings

Per Serving
Calories: 127
Calories from fat: 61
Total fat: 7 g
Saturated fat: 1 g
Cholesterol: 0 mg
Sodium: 36 mg
Carbohydrates: 17 g
Fiber: 3 g
Sugar: 9 g
Protein: 1 g
Vitamin A: 104% DV
Vitamin C: 11% DV
Calcium: 11% DV
Iron: 6% DV

Marinated Parsnips

I feel like parsnips often get left behind in favor of their close cousin, the carrot. If you have not tried parsnips before, you should give them a shot. They are sweet and earthy. I actually find them sweeter than carrots and enjoy them in salads and soups alike. This recipe is mildly anti-inflammatory.

2 pounds parsnips, peeled and cut on a diagonal in 1-inch pieces
1 large onion, peeled and sliced into thin rings
1 large green pepper, sliced into match sticks
1 can tomato soup
½ cup honey
¾ cup apple cider vinegar
⅓ cup olive oil
Salt and pepper to taste

Bring a large pot of water to a boil. Add the parsnips and a pinch of salt. Bring to a boil, reduce the heat, and simmer for 10 minutes.

Drain parsnips and cool.

In a large bowl, combine the parsnips, green pepper, and onion rings. Set aside.

Combine soup, honey vinegar, oil, and salt and pepper to taste in a medium saucepan over medium-high heat. Bring to a boil.

Pour the hot mixture over the vegetables. Cool, cover, and chill in refrigerator overnight. Serve cold or at room temperature.

Free of
casein, corn, dairy, eggs, fish, gluten

Prep time
15 minutes

Total time
1¼ hours

Makes
4 servings

Per Serving
Calories: 310
Calories from fat: 172
Total Fat: 20 g
Saturated Fat: 3 g
Cholesterol: 0 mg
Sodium: 200 mg
Carbohydrates: 86 g
Fiber: 9 g
Sugar: 20 g
Protein: 3 g
Vitamin A: 31% DV
Vitamin C: 156% DV
Calcium: 9% DV
Iron: 14% DV

Sun-Dried Tomato Grilled Eggplant

This recipe is inspired by my friend Phil, who is a very good pizza maker. I decided to turn the toppings he loves into something I could eat, since gluten-free me cannot eat "normal" pizza. This is what I came up with. It makes a great side dish. Serve it over brown rice or millet. For extra protein, you may also add ½ cup adzuki beans. This recipe is moderately anti-inflammatory.

1 eggplant, cut into chunks, unpeeled
¼ cup extra-virgin olive oil
Salt and pepper to taste
½ cup of chopped sun-dried tomatoes
2 roasted red peppers, chopped
12 leaves basil, chopped
½ cup pine nuts, toasted (optional)

Heat a grill pan on an outdoor grill to high heat. Combine the eggplant with the olive oil in a medium-size bowl and toss to coat. Add salt and pepper.

Grill the eggplant for 5–8 minutes on each side.

Return the eggplant to the bowl. Add the sun-dried tomatoes, red peppers, basil, and toasted pine nuts.

Free of
casein, corn, dairy, eggs, fish, gluten

Prep time
10 minutes

Total time
20 minutes

Makes
4 servings

Per Serving
Calories: 261
Calories from fat: 226
Total fat: 26 g
Saturated fat: 3 g
Cholesterol: 0 mg
Sodium: 135 mg
Carbohydrates: 7 g
Fiber: 2 g
Sugar: 4 g
Protein: 3 g
Vitamin A: 21% DV
Vitamin C: 58% DV
Iron: 8% DV
Calcium: 2% DV

Portobello Steaks

Portobellos are beefy and delicious. I love them!

4 large Portobello mushrooms

2 tablespoons olive oil

2 tablespoons balsamic vinegar

3 teaspoons dried oregano

1 teaspoon dried rosemary

Salt and pepper to taste

Preheat oven to 350°F.

Remove the stems from the mushrooms. Wash both the tops and stems.

Mix oil, vinegar, oregano, and rosemary in a dish.

Put the mushroom tops and stems in a shallow baking dish. Pour the oil mixture over the mushrooms and bake for 30 minutes.

Free of
casein, corn, dairy, eggs, fish, gluten

Prep time
5 minutes

Total time
35 minutes

Makes
4 servings

Per Serving
Calories: 112
Calories from fat: 68
Total fat: 8 g
Saturated fat: 1 g
Cholesterol: 0 mg
Sodium: 14 mg
Carbohydrates: 8 g
Fiber: 3 g
Sugar: 1 g
Protein: 5 g
Vitamin A: 1% DV
Vitamin C: 1% DV
Calcium: 2% DV
Iron: 6% DV

Tomato Simmered String Beans

My favorite Greek restaurant makes this, so I had to figure out how to make it on my own. Here is my version, and I think it's dead on.

1 pound string beans, rinsed and stems removed
2 cloves garlic, minced
3 tablespoons olive oil
1 14-ounce can fire-roasted tomatoes
½ cup toasted pine nuts
Juice of ½ lemon

Heat the olive oil in a large skillet. Add the green beans and garlic and sauté for 10 minutes. Add the fire-roasted tomatoes and continue to cook until heated through. Sprinkle pine nuts and lemon juice on top to serve.

Free of
casein, corn, dairy, eggs, fish, gluten

Prep time
5 minutes

Total time
20 minutes

Makes
4 servings

Per Serving
Calories: 298
Calories from fat: 192
Total fat: 22 g
Saturated fat: 2 g
Cholesterol: 0 mg
Sodium: 265 mg
Carbohydrates: 24 g
Fiber: 7 g
Sugar: 2 g
Protein: 7 g
Vitamin A: 39% DV
Vitamin C: 63% DV
Calcium: 10% DV
Iron: 25% DV

These salads are designed for an on-the-go lunch. You can pair the salad with piece of fruit and some healthy whole-grain crackers in a bento box. These salads avoid potential allergens, so they do not contain traditional mayonnaise. There's an added bonus: These dressings have no egg and therefore do not need to be refrigerated, making them ideal for a barbecue or picnic.

Carrot and Raisin Salad

My son is in love with carrots, so I began making this for his nursery-school snack. It's tasty, simple, and packed with vitamin A!

1 pound carrots, grated
⅔ cup raisins
1½ cups freshly squeezed orange juice
1 tablespoon freshly grated ginger root

Soak raisins in orange juice for 1 hour. Overnight is also fine.

Mix all ingredients in a bowl and marinate for 1 hour or overnight.

Free of
casein, corn, dairy, eggs, fish, gluten

Prep time
10 minutes

Total time
70 minutes

Makes
4 servings

Per Serving
Calories: 112
Calories from fat: 3
Total fat: less than 1 g
Saturated fat: 0 g
Cholesterol: 0 mg
Sodium: 19 mg
Carbohydrates: 28 g
Fiber: 2 g
Sugar: 9 g
Protein: 1 g
Vitamin A: 45% DV
Vitamin C: 80% DV
Calcium: 2% DV
Iron: 5% DV

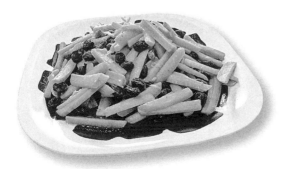

Far-Out Fruit Salad

This fruit salad is great for breakfast, paired with lunch, or served as a nice dessert with dark chocolate chips!

1 pear, peeled, cored, cubed
1 small apple, chopped
1½ cup cubed pineapple
¼ cup shredded carrots
½ cup chopped celery
¼ cup raisins
⅓ cup walnuts
⅓ cup Enriching Eggless Mayo (see recipe on page 255)
¼ cup lemon juice

Combine the fruit, vegetables, raisins, and walnuts in a large bowl. Stir the lemon juice into the mayonnaise and stir. Pour mix over the salad and blend well. Store in refrigerator until ready to serve.

Free of
casein, corn, dairy, eggs, fish, gluten

Prep time
20 minutes

Total time
20 minutes

Makes
4 servings

Per Serving
Calories: 224
Calories from fat: 108
Total fat: 12 g
Saturated fat: 1 g
Cholesterol: 0 mg
Sodium: 160 mg
Carbohydrates: 29 g
Fiber: 4 g
Sugar: 14 g
Protein: 3 g
Vitamin A: 5% DV
Vitamin C: 67% DV
Calcium: 4% DV
Iron: 5% DV

Cheerfully Cherry Pecan Salad

I love cherries when they are in season. They are sweet, with a touch of tartness. Nutrition-wise, they are very high in vitamin C, making them a superb anti-cancer fruit. Since those who have IBD are at a greater risk for colon cancer, this recipe is particularly helpful in maintaining health. Take advantage of this salad when cherries are in season.

2 heads romaine lettuce, chopped
1 cup baby arugula, tightly packed
1 cup unsweetened dried cherries
1 cup raw pecans
½ red onion, chopped
½ cup cherry juice
½ cup balsamic vinegar
Sprinkle Parmesan cheese (optional)

Combine the first 5 ingredients in a large bowl. Blend the cherry juice and balsamic vinegar in a small bowl. Pour over the salad and toss. Serve immediately with a dash of Parmesan, if desired.

Free of
casein, corn, dairy, eggs, fish, gluten

Prep time
10 minutes

Total time
12 minutes

Makes
4 servings

Per Serving
Calories: 258
Calories from fat: 166
Total fat: 20 g
Saturated fat: 2 g
Cholesterol: 0 mg
Sodium: 16 mg
Carbohydrates: 19 g
Fiber: 5 g
Sugar: 11 g
Protein: 4 g
Vitamin A: 89% DV
Vitamin C: 709% DV
Calcium: 6% DV
Iron: 10% DV

Tangy Tuna Salad

This tuna salad is different than your traditional mayonnaise-based salad. The dill pickle is the secret ingredient! Use on gluten-free whole-grain bread or with gluten-free crackers. Or serve over a bed of fresh arugula. This dish is moderately anti-inflammatory.

1 6-ounce can light chunk tuna, packed in water, drained
1 dill pickle, finely chopped
¼ cup diced roasted red pepper
¼ cup chopped fresh parsley
3 tablespoons olive oil
2 tablespoons mustard
Salt to taste

Put the drained tuna, pickle, pepper, and parsley in a mixing bowl. Combine well.

Put the olive oil in a small bowl and whisk in the mustard. Add salt to taste. Pour over the tuna mixture and combine.

Free of
casein, corn, dairy, eggs, fish, gluten

Prep time
5 minutes

Total time
7 minutes

Makes
4 servings

Per Serving
Calories: 134
Calories from fat: 101
Total Fat: 11 g
Saturated fat: 2 g
Cholesterol: 8 mg
Sodium: 355 mg
Carbohydrates: 3 g
Fiber: 1 g
Sugar: 1 g
Protein: 6 g
Vitamin A: 35% DV
Vitamin C: 57% DV
Calcium: 3% DV
Iron: 5% DV

Kiwi Avocado Salad

Creamy avocado and sweet, tangy kiwi provide a nice combination in this side salad. I like to serve this with a turkey sandwich with arugula and mustard on crusty gluten-free bread. It makes an excellent lunch.

2 kiwis, peeled and chopped
1 avocado, peeled, stone removed, and chopped
1 scallion, chopped on an angle
Salt to taste
2 teaspoons fresh lime juice
Pinch of red pepper flake

Combine the kiwi, avocado, and scallion in a small bowl. Sprinkle with lime juice and red pepper flakes. Chill or serve immediately at room temperature.

Free of
casein, corn, dairy, eggs, fish, gluten

Prep time
10 minutes

Total time
10 minutes

Makes
4 servings

Per Serving
Calories: 102
Calories from fat: 51
Total fat: 6 g
Saturated fat: 1 g
Cholesterol: 0 mg
Sodium: 5 mg
Carbohydrates: 12 g
Fiber: 5 g
Sugar: 6 g
Protein: 2 g
Vitamin A: 6% DV
Vitamin C: 91% DV
Calcium: 3% DV
Iron: 3% DV

Mango-Strawberry Salad

Tropical and full of vitamin C, this fruit salad is versatile: It fits into breakfast, lunch, or dinner or can be eaten as a snack. This dish is moderately anti-inflammatory.

½ cup extra virgin olive oil

1 teaspoon lemon juice

½ teaspoon dry mustard

½ teaspoon onion powder

½ teaspoon garlic powder

⅛ teaspoon chili powder

⅛ teaspoon salt

2 cups cubed mango

2 cups sliced strawberries

1 cup cubed pineapple

1 small head romaine lettuce, cleaned and chopped

¼ cup sliced almonds or walnuts (optional)

Put the olive oil in a small bowl and whisk in the lemon juice, mustard, onion powder, garlic powder, chili powder, and salt.

Put the fruit and romaine lettuce in a salad bowl. Pour dressing over salad and sprinkle with nuts if desired.

Free of
casein, corn, dairy, eggs, fish, gluten

Prep time
15 minutes

Total time
20 minutes

Makes
6 servings

Per Serving
Calories: 273
Calories from fat: 191
Total fat: 22 g
Saturated fat: 3 g
Cholesterol: 0 mg
Sodium: 12 mg
Carbohydrates: 20 g
Fiber: 4 g
Sugar: 14 g
Protein: 3 g
Vitamin A: 40% DV
Vitamin C: 110% DV
Calcium: 5% DV
Iron: 6% DV

Most people with IBD think dessert is out. While sugar is not compatible with IBD, there are many treats you can still enjoy that won't cause a flare-up. This is why I replaced refined sugars with natural sweeteners in the *IBD Healing Plan and Recipe Book*. You'll see that I even sneak vegetables into some of these desserts, which is an excellent way to add more nutrients into your diet.

Just a note about the recipes: Most of the time a sweet vegetable purée will work as a substitute for eggs. Be creative as you try these recipes and see where you can add more nutrient-dense foods. If you don't have time to cook and purée vegetables, use a high-quality, organic baby food. It is an excellent time-saving alternative.

Nutty Natural Caramel Balls

Dates are completely underrated, in my opinion. I love using them as a healthy sugar substitute in recipes. These treats contain a lot of anti-inflammatory healthy fats, thanks to the coconut flakes, which are loaded with omega-3 fatty acids. Eliminate the walnuts if you are experiencing a flare-up.

1 cup dates
1 cup unsweetened coconut flakes
1 cup chopped raw almonds or walnuts

Purée the dates in a food processor and form into bite-size balls.

Combine the coconut and almonds. Roll date balls in the coconut–almond mixture to coat.

Refrigerate for 2 hours to harden. Store in an airtight container.

Free of
casein, corn, dairy, eggs, fish, gluten

Prep time
10 minutes

Total time
2 hours and 10 minutes

Makes
16 small balls

Per Ball
Calories: 98
Calories from fat: 51
Total fat: 6 g
Saturated fat: 2 g
Cholesterol: 0 mg
Sodium: 18 mg
Carbohydrates: 10 g
Fiber: 2 g
Sugars: 7 g
Protein: 2 g
Vitamin A: 0% DV
Vitamin C: 0% DV
Calcium: 2% DV
Iron: 3% DV

Pumpkin Quinoa Cookies

The pumpkin and maple syrup adds a sweetness to this cookie that is wonderful! When taste testing these cookies, my other half claimed they are like a cross between a donut and a pumpkin spice cake. The quinoa adds protein and vitamins B and E.

1 cup gluten-free baking mix

1 teaspoon pumpkin pie spice or 1 teaspoon cinnamon, with a pinch of nutmeg

½ teaspoon baking soda

½ teaspoon salt

1 cup maple syrup

½ cup melted coconut oil or soy butter

¼ cup puréed sweet potato

2 vanilla beans, scraped with the seeds discarded

½ cup puréed pumpkin

2 cups quinoa flakes

1 cup dried cranberries or raisins (optional)

Preheat oven to 350°F.

Line two cookie sheets with parchment paper, taping if necessary, to keep it from moving around.

Combine flour, pumpkin pie spice, baking soda, and salt in a medium bowl.

Free of
casein, corn, dairy, eggs, fish, gluten, nuts

Prep time
10 minutes

Total time
32 minutes

Makes
2 dozen cookies

Per Cookie
Calories: 287
Calories from fat: 78
Total fat: 9 g
Saturated fat: 6 g
Cholesterol: 0 mg
Sodium: 109 mg
Carbohydrates: 48 g
Fiber: 3 g
Sugars: 23 g
Protein: 4 g
Vitamin A: 40% DV
Vitamin C: 1% DV
Calcium: 4% DV
Iron: 11% DV

Put the maple syrup and coconut oil in a large mixing bowl and mix with an electric mixer at medium speed until light and fluffy, about 5 minutes.

Add sweet potato purée and beat in vanilla beans, discarding the seeds and stem. Reduce to low speed and add pumpkin. Beat until blended. Add flour mixture until just blended. Stir in quinoa flakes and cranberries and incorporate well. Form dough into rounded teaspoonfuls and place 2 inches apart on the prepared cookie sheets.

Bake for 12 minutes, or until golden brown. Cool.

Virgin Piña Colada Smoothie Pops

This is one of my summer favorites! It's cooling and refreshing—and also reminiscent of one of my favorite cocktails. You get the added benefit of pineapple's anti-inflammatory qualities, thanks to its high concentration of bromelain. These pops are the exact opposite of their alcoholic cousin, as they come with all of the flavor but none of the inflammatory risk you get from drinking alcohol.

1 can coconut milk
1 fresh pineapple, peeled, cored, and roughly chopped
1 cup orange juice
Juice from ½ lemon
2 tablespoons honey

Combine all the ingredients in blender and blend at high speed for 3 minutes. Pour into ice pop molds. Freeze for 2 hours.

Free of
casein, corn, dairy, eggs, fish, gluten, nuts

Prep time
5 minutes

Total time
2 hours

Makes
6 pops

Per Serving
Calories: 209
Calories from fat: 122
Total fat: 15 g
Saturated fat: 13 g
Cholesterol: 0 mg
Sodium: 10 mg
Carbohydrates: 22 g
Fiber: 3 g
Sugars: 13 g
Protein: 2 g
Vitamin A: 1% DV
Vitamin C: 44% DV
Calcium: 2% DV
Iron: 7% DV

Yummy, Healthy Onion Rings

I find I enjoy this healthy version of onion rings much more than the traditional way of making them, which is usually covered with gluten and deep fried. The ingredient that makes this recipe so good is actually the rice-flour bread crumbs. Gluten-free bread-crumbs are very light and fluffy and make for a great crust when baked! They taste just like the real thing without the grease.

2 large onions, peeled and cut into ¼-inch slices
½ cup puréed spinach, spinach baby food, or 6 tablespoons warm water plus 2 tablespoons ground flaxseed
1½ cups gluten-free bread crumbs
Salt and pepper to taste
Olive oil spray to coat pan

Preheat oven to 375°F.

Coat a large baking sheet with olive oil spray.

Put the spinach purée or flaxseed/water mixture in a large bowl. Add the onions gently to bowl and coat well.

Spread the bread crumbs over a large plate or sheet of parchment paper. Individually coat the onions evenly with the crumbs, making sure to shake off any excess.

Place the onions in a single layer across baking sheet, sprinkle with salt and pepper, and bake for 15 minutes, or until golden brown. They can be eaten plain or served with tartar, ketchup, or barbecue sauce.

Free of
casein, corn, dairy, eggs, fish, gluten, nuts

Prep time
5 minutes

Total time
20 minutes

Makes about
2 dozen rings

Per Ring
Calories: 9
Calories from fat: 2
Total fat: less than 1 g
Saturated fat: 0 g
Cholesterol: 4 mg
Sodium: 8 mg
Carbohydrates: 2 g
Fiber: 0 g
Sugars: 1 g
Protein: 2 g
Vitamin A: 1% DV
Vitamin C: 1% DV
Calcium: 1% DV
Iron: 3% DV

Zesty Zucchini or Eggplant Sticks

Same concept as the onion ring. These zucchini sticks are great as an appetizer, for a light lunch with a salad, or as a take-along to a potluck party.

2 medium zucchinis
½ cup of spinach purée or 6 tablespoons warm water plus 2 tablespoons ground flaxseed
1½ cups gluten-free bread crumbs
Salt and pepper to taste
Olive oil spray

Optional toppings:
½ cup chopped toasted walnuts
1 teaspoon salt
1 cup tomato sauce

Preheat oven to 375°F. Coat a large baking sheet with 1–2 teaspoons olive oil.

Cut the zucchini in half, lengthwise. Then slice each half widthwise. Cut into ¼ inch-thick sticks. Set aside.

Put the spinach or flaxseed/water mixture in a medium bowl. Add the zucchini and toss to coat well.

Spread the bread crumbs out over a large plate

Free of
casein, corn, dairy, eggs, fish, gluten, nuts

Prep time
10 minutes

Total time
25 minutes

Makes about
2 dozen zucchini sticks or 2 servings

Per Serving (Without Toppings)
Calories: 151
Calories from fat: 74
Total fat: 9 g
Saturated fat: 1 g
Cholesterol: 8 g
Sodium: 266 mg
Carbohydrates: 15 g
Fiber: 3 g
Sugars: 6 g
Protein: 4 g
Vitamin A: 38% DV
Vitamin C: 11% DV
Calcium: 9% DV
Iron: 6% DV

or sheet of parchment paper. Remove the zucchini sticks from the coating and press into the bread crumbs to coat them evenly, making sure to shake off excess.

Place the zucchini sticks in a single layer across baking sheet, sprinkle with salt and pepper, and bake for 15 minutes, or until golden brown. If using cheese topping, combine walnuts and salt. Top zucchini sticks with mixture just before serving. Serve with tomato sauce for dipping.

Cheery Cherry Almond Cupcookie

I always bring this marriage of a cookie and a cupcake dessert to parties, and it is always very popular. You can substitute whipped soy cream or puréed frozen bananas for the glaze.

⅔ cup agave nectar

¾ cup toasted almonds

4 tablespoons softened soy butter

¼ teaspoon salt

¼ cup rice milk

Juice of one lemon

¾ cup unsweetened apple sauce

½ teaspoon almond extract

1⅓ cup gluten-free baking mix

½ teaspoon gluten-free baking powder

2 cups (about 2 15-ounce cans) unsweetened, pitted dark cherries, halved with juice reserved

½ teaspoon guar gum

To make the cherry juice glaze:

1 cup reserved cherry juice

¼ cup arrowroot starch or cornstarch

½ cup agave nectar

½ teaspoon almond extract (optional)

Preheat oven to 375°F.

Prepare bake ware: The cookies can be baked in eight 6-ounce ramekins, large or regular muffin pans, or in an 8 x 8-inch baking dish. Use melted coconut oil to grease the bake ware. If using individual ramekins, set them on a large baking sheet.

Free of
gluten, eggs, soy, dairy, casein, corn

Prep time
10 minutes

Total time
40 minutes

Makes
12 cookies or 6 servings

Per Serving (2 Cookies)
Calories: 225
Calories from fat: 70
Total fat: 8 g
Saturated fat: 1 g
Cholesterol: 0 mg
Sodium: 49 mg
Carbohydrates: 37 g
Fiber: 3 g
Sugars: 22 g
Protein: 4 g
Vitamin A: 9% DV
Vitamin C: 693% DV
Calcium: 4% DV
Iron: 5% DV

To make the cookies: Put the agave nectar, ¼ cup of the toasted almonds, butter, and salt in a food processor and pulse until the nuts are finely ground and the mixture is well combined.

Add the rice milk, lemon, applesauce, and almond extract and pulse until the mixture is smooth. Add the baking mix and baking powder and pulse to combine. Pour the batter into a mixing bowl and fold in the prepared cherries and guar gum. Fill ramekins or muffin cups about ⅔ full with batter or add all to cake pan. Coarsely chop remaining ½ cup toasted almonds and scatter nuts on top of the batter.

Bake for about 30 minutes, or until done.

To make cherry juice glaze: Pour reserved cherry juice in a medium saucepan over medium heat. Add arrowroot or cornstarch and whisk to dissolve. Add agave and whisk until the mixture thickens. Remove from heat and whisk in almond extract, if using.

Banana Cherry Fruit Squares

One of my son's friends was surprised that I knew how to make "fruit roll-ups" at home, yet they are so easy. Both kids and adults love them. There is no added sugar—the fruit itself is sweet enough—which makes these much healthier than commercial brands.

2 bananas, large
1 cup frozen cherries, thawed, juice reserved
1 teaspoon lemon juice
Water as needed

Preheat oven to 275°F.

Purée the cherries in a blender with the reserved cherry juice and lemon juice, adding water as needed to make a smooth purée.

Pour the mixture onto a baking sheet fitted with parchment paper or coated with cooking spray. Be sure to spread very flat, or fruit squares will be gummy. Bake for 60 minutes. Leave fruit in the oven to dry for at least 8–10 hours or overnight.

Once dry, place a large piece of parchment paper over the top of the fruit to cover. Using a cookie cutter, cut into 12 squares. Store in a plastic container.

Note: You can substitute the cherries for 2 cups of puréed fruit of any variety.

Free of
casein, corn, dairy, eggs, fish, gluten, nuts

Prep time
10 minutes

Total time
45 minutes

Makes
12 squares

Per Square
Calories: 42
Calories from fat: 1
Total fat: less than 1 g
Saturated fat: 0 g
Cholesterol: 0 mg
Sodium: 0 mg
Carbohydrates: 11 g
Fiber: 1 g
Sugars: 6 g
Protein: 1 g
Vitamin A: 1% DV
Vitamin C: 10% DV
Calcium: 0% DV
Iron: 1% DV

Dairy-Free Whipped Rice Cream

When I went dairy free I really missed whipped cream. Then I came up with this rice-based substitute. It is light and airy, and I find it to be sinfully delicious.

½ cup rice milk

1 teaspoon vanilla

½ cup melted coconut oil

2 tablespoons maple syrup

Pinch of salt

2 egg whites, beaten to stiff peaks (optional)

Put the milk and vanilla in a blender and blend, gradually adding the coconut oil, until the mixture becomes thick. If needed, add more coconut oil. Incorporate honey and salt. If you tolerate eggs, add the beaten egg for a thicker consistency.

Free of
casein, corn, dairy, eggs, fish, gluten, nuts

Prep time
10 minutes

Total time
10 minutes

Makes
1 cup (8 2-tablespoon servings)

Per Serving
Calories: 104
Calories from fat: 81
Total fat: 9 g
Saturated fat: 8 g
Cholesterol: 0 mg
Sodium: 10 mg
Carbohydrates: 4 g
Fiber: 0 g
Sugars: 2 g
Protein: 1 g
Vitamin A: 0% DV
Vitamin C: 0% DV
Calcium: 0% DV
Iron: 0% DV

Mighty Mango Banana Cream Machine

Tropical mango is wonderful in flavor and contains a good amount of immune-protecting vitamin C. This dessert is great for when you are having a flare-up; I find the vitamin C really gives me a good boost!

2 cups rice milk

2 tablespoons arrowroot

2–3 medium mangoes, about 1 pound, peeled, seeded, and diced

1 whole pineapple, peeled, cored, and chopped

½ medium-sized papaya, peeled, seeded, and chopped

1 large banana

½ cup orange juice

Juice from 1 lime

3 tablespoons honey, maple syrup, or agave nectar

1 mango, cut into wedges

1 lime, cut into wedges

Free of
casein, corn, dairy, eggs, fish, gluten, nuts

Prep time
10 minutes

Total time
15 minutes

Makes
6 servings

Per Serving
Calories: 99
Calories from fat: 3
Total fat: less than 1 g
Saturated fat: 0 g
Cholesterol: 0 mg
Sodium: 2 mg
Carbohydrates: 25 g
Fiber: 2 g
Sugars: 17 g
Protein: 1 g
Vitamin A: 9% DV
Vitamin C: 60% DV
Calcium: 1% DV
Iron: 2% DV

Heat the milk to boiling over medium-low heat. Meanwhile, mix the arrowroot with 1–2 tablespoons of water in a bowl, until it forms a thick paste. Remove the milk from heat and add arrowroot mixture, stirring until the mixture thickens. Set aside to cool.

While the milk is cooling, purée the mango, pineapple, papaya, orange juice, lime juice, and banana in a blender until smooth and creamy.

Combine fruit purée, milk, and sweetener. Spoon into individual bowls and chill.

Serve with slices of fresh mango and a slice of lime.

Brown Rice Pudding

Love pudding? Then you will simply love this one, which is equally good as a dessert as it is for breakfast. I like adding grated apple for sweetness, and one day, I decided to add some carrot for more sweetness and crunch. It turned out to be a family hit. This recipe can be made in advance. Just reheat it on the stovetop and serve.

1 cup brown rice
1 cup coconut, soy, almond, or rice milk
½ cup pecans or almonds
1 gala apple, peeled, cored, and grated
½ cup raisins or other dried fruit
½ cup shredded carrots
3 tablespoons maple syrup
2 tablespoons vanilla extract
1 teaspoon cinnamon
Salt to taste

Cook rice according to package instructions.

Once rice has finished cooking, stir the remaining ingredients into the warm rice and serve hot.

Variation: Change the flavor to your liking. Add a small amount of chocolate syrup or chocolate soy milk for a chocolate "Rice Krispies" cereal taste. Change the fruit to cherries and substitute a different type of nut. Use dried cranberries instead of raisins. Or add a cup of sunflower seeds or pumpkin seeds, in addition to the dried fruit.

Free of
gluten, dairy, casein, soy, nuts, sugar, eggs, fish

Prep time
15 minutes

Total time
1 hour

Makes
6 servings

Per Serving
Calories: 248
Calories from fat: 69
Total fat: 8 g
Saturated fat: 2 g
Cholesterol: 0 mg
Sodium: 32 mg
Carbohydrates: 41 g
Fiber: 5 g
Sugars: 11 g
Protein: 3 g
Vitamin A: 85% DV
Vitamin C: 4% DV
Calcium: 6% DV
Iron: 9% DV

Mock Cook 'n' Serve Vanilla Pudding

Sweet potato thickens this pudding into a creamy consistency while lending a hint of sweetness.

2 15-ounce cans coconut milk
¾ cup agave nectar
¼ cup puréed sweet potato
The seeds from the insides of 3 vanilla beans
2 tablespoons brown rice flour
Pinch salt

Put coconut milk, agave, sweet potato, and vanilla beans in a medium saucepan over high heat and bring to a boil, stirring constantly. Add flour and salt. Turn heat down to simmer. Continue cooking, stirring constantly, for about 5–8 minutes, or until mixture has thickened. Serve pudding warm or at room temperature.

Tip: For extra vanilla flavor, add the whole bean into the pudding while cooking and remove before service.

Free of
casein, corn, dairy, eggs, fish, gluten, nuts

Prep time
5 minutes

Total time
20 minutes

Makes
6 servings

Per Serving
Calories: 178
Calories from fat: 26
Total fat: 3 g
Saturated fat: 3 g
Cholesterol: 0 mg
Sodium: 11 mg
Carbohydrates: 35 g
Fiber: 0 g
Sugars: 31 g
Protein: 1 g
Vitamin A: 21% DV
Vitamin C: 0% DV
Calcium: 5% DV
Iron: 3% DV

Frozen Dark Chocolate Banana Pops

This may just be my personal favorite recipe in this book. It is not only easy, it is guiltless, as dark chocolate contains a bounty of good-for-you phytonutrients and bananas are rich in important minerals. I prefer Green & Black's Organic Dark Chocolate with Hazelnuts and Currants, but any chocolate will do as long as it is dark. This recipe works well with blueberries, strawberries, and pineapple as well.

2 large bananas
2 3½-ounce bars dark chocolate, coarsely
  chopped

Peel the bananas and place them in a freezer bag or freezer-safe plastic container. Let set for 2 hours.

Put the chocolate in the top of a double broiler over medium-low heat and whisk around until the chocolate melts. You can also use the microwave to melt the chocolate, about 3 minutes on medium-high heat.

Place the frozen bananas in the melted chocolate to coat. Place the bananas back into the container and freeze for 2 more hours, or until the chocolate is hard. Cut in two and serve.

Free of
casein, corn, dairy, eggs, fish, gluten, nuts

Prep time
5 minutes

Total time
4 hours

Makes
4 servings

Per ½ Banana
Calories: 201
Calories from fat: 98
Total fat: 11 g
Saturated fat: 6g
Cholesterol: 1 mg
Sodium: 6 mg
Carbohydrates: 24 g
Fiber: 8 g
Sugars: 13 g
Protein: 2 g
Vitamin A: 2% DV
Vitamin C: 16% DV
Calcium: 4% DV
Iron: 12% DV

These condiments will get your mouth watering faster than you can say, "dip." Use the dips as an accompaniment to crackers and crudités, or even as a complement to a wrap. In addition to using them on salads, the dressings can be used as marinades or as toppings for wraps and sandwiches.

Totally Tofu Sour Cream

This recipe is very close to traditional dairy sour cream! You can find powdered soymilk in most health-food stores or online. This recipe is anti-inflammatory.

5 tablespoons powdered soymilk
1 tablespoon lemon juice
1 tablespoon red wine vinegar
1 cup crumbled tofu

Put all ingredients in blender and whip until smooth. It will keep, refrigerated, for about a week or so.

Free of
casein, corn, dairy, eggs, fish, gluten, nuts

Prep time
3 minutes

Total time
5 minutes

Makes about
1⅓ cups
(32 2-teaspoon servings)

Per Serving
Calories: 4
Calories from fat: 1
Total fat: less than 1 g
Saturated fat: 0 g
Cholesterol: 0 mg
Sodium: 0 mg
Carbohydrates: 0 g
Fiber: 0 g
Sugars: 0 g
Protein: 0 g
Vitamin A: 1% DV
Vitamin C: 3% DV
Calcium: 3% DV
Iron: 1% DV

Nana's Vegetable Dip

My grandmother made some of the absolute best food on earth. I was lucky enough to inherit her huge recipe box, and this is a recipe card I pull out often. It is carefully written with her shaky handwriting. The smoky character from the curry, blended with the sweetness from the ketchup, make it an ideal complement to chopped veggies and salads.

1½ cups Enriching Eggless Mayo (see recipe on page 255)

2 tablespoons ketchup

2 tablespoons honey

1 teaspoon curry powder

1 tablespoon dried onion

1 teaspoon lemon juice

1 dash of Tabasco sauce (optional)

Salt and pepper to taste

Blend all ingredients in a medium bowl with a wire whisk. Store in the refrigerator.

Free of
casein, corn, dairy, eggs, gluten, nuts

Prep time
10 minutes

Total time
10 minutes

Makes about
2 cups

Per Teaspoon
Calories: 3
Calories from fat: 0
Total fat: 0 g
Saturated Fat: 0 g
Cholesterol: 0 mg
Sodium: 0 mg
Carbohydrates: 1 g
Fiber: 0 g
Sugars: 0 g
Protein: 0 g
Vitamin A: 1% DV
Vitamin C: 0% DV
Calcium: 1% DV
Iron: 2% DV

Marvelous Maple BBQ Dressing

This is a modified version of my favorite dressing from my favorite cook, Rachel Ray. It's a great way to get kids to eat salad because they love the sweet and tangy flavor of the dressing. The dressing is loaded with lycopene from the maple syrup.

½ cup orange juice
½ cup pure maple syrup
½ cup barbecue sauce
1 teaspoon grainy mustard
¼ cup extra virgin olive oil
Salt and pepper to taste

Mix the first 4 ingredients together with a wire whisk and then slowly incorporate the olive oil. Season to taste.

Free of
casein, corn, dairy, eggs, gluten, nuts

Prep time
5 minutes

Total time
5 minutes

Makes about
2 cups (8 ¼-cup servings)

Per Serving
Calories: 93
Calories from fat: 40
Total fat: 5 g
Saturated fat: 1 g
Cholesterol: 0 mg
Sodium: 118 mg
Carbohydrates: 13 g
Fiber: 0 g
Sugars: 12 g
Protein: 0 g
Vitamin A: 0% DV
Vitamin C: 10% DV
Calcium: 1% DV
Iron: 2% DV

Simply Simple Avocado Dip

My son's paternal grandmother is an expert on all Indonesian foods. One of her favorite ingredients is avocados, and she uses them in everything! Simple, elegant, and creamy, avocados have cooling properties that are quite soothing to the digestive tract.

1 large avocado, pitted and peeled
Juice of 1 lime
1 tomato, diced
2 scallions, white and green parts, chopped
Dash or 2 Tabasco sauce
Salt and pepper to taste

Mash avocado with a fork or in a food processor until very smooth and mix it generously with the lime juice to protect its color. Add the tomato, scallions, and Tabasco, and add salt and pepper to taste. Blend.

Free of
casein, corn, dairy, eggs, fish, gluten, nuts

Prep time
5 minutes

Total time
5 minutes

Makes
12 servings

Per Serving
Calories: 26
Calories from fat: 16
Total fat: 2 g
Saturated fat: 0 g
Cholesterol: 0 mg
Sodium: 6 mg
Carbohydrates: 2 g
Fiber: 1 g
Sugars: 1 g
Protein: 1 g
Vitamin A: 5% DV
Vitamin C: 11% DV
Calcium: 0% DV
Iron: 1% DV

Nana's Irresistible French Dressing

My Nana would always make this dressing to accompany her traditional Sunday salads. I have modified it slightly with flaxseeds for some added omega-3 fatty acids. It is crisp and smooth and has just the right level of tanginess.

1 14-ounce can tomato soup
¼ cup extra virgin olive oil
¼ cup flaxseed oil
½ cup of honey
1 small onion, diced
1 4-ounce can pimentos
¾ teaspoon dry mustard
1¼ teaspoons salt

Combine all ingredients together in an air-tight glass jar. Shake to combine.

Refrigerate for up to 2 weeks.

Free of
casein, corn, dairy, eggs, fish, gluten, nuts

Prep time
5 minutes

Total time
5 minutes

Makes about
2½ cups
(12 3-teaspoon servings)

Per Serving
Calories: 226
Calories from fat: 160
Total fat: 18 g
Saturated fat: 2 g
Cholesterol: 0 mg
Sodium: 83 mg
Total carbohydrate: 18 g
Fiber: 3 g
Sugars: 14 g
Protein: 1 g
Vitamin A: 6% DV
Vitamin C: 14% DV
Calcium: 14% DV
Iron: 5% DV

Comfort Cranberry Sauce

My mom and I have been making this cranberry sauce for the past few years. My family knows it will always be on the table every holiday, and they always look forward to it. When I changed my diet years ago, I had to start making my own cranberry sauce, because I love it so much. Give this a try next Thanksgiving! Your cranberry sauce fans will relish it!

4 cups fresh cranberries, about 1 pound

1½ cups agave nectar

1 cup water

1 whole orange, unpeeled, seeds removed, diced

1 cup diced fresh pineapple

½ cup chopped walnuts (optional)

Sprinkle of pumpkin pie spice

Wash and pick over cranberries. Discard the ones that are not firm.

Bring the agave and water to a boil in a large saucepan over high heat Add cranberries, oranges, and pumpkin pie spice.

Simmer over a high flame, stirring frequently, until berries pop open.

Add the pineapple and walnuts and blend.

Cool and serve.

Free of
casein, corn, dairy, eggs, fish, gluten, nuts

Prep time
10 minutes

Total time
15 minutes

Makes about
4 cups (8 ½-cup servings)

Per Serving
Calories: 101
Calories from fat: 54
Total fat: 6 g
Saturated fat: 1 g
Cholesterol: 0 mg
Sodium: 1 mg
Carbohydrate: 11 g
Fiber: 3 g
Sugars: 4 g
Protein: 2 g
Vitamin A: 1% DV
Vitamin C: 36% DV
Calcium: 2% DV
Iron: 3% DV

Creamy Peanut Sauce

This recipe is courtesy of my son's paternal grandmother, Nuri Hannan, who hails from Indonesia. She makes the best peanut sauce I have ever tasted. Make sure to use organic peanuts to avoid reactions from genetically modified ones.

1 cup peanut butter (or cashew butter if peanuts not tolerated)
¼ cup orange juice
1 tablespoon toasted sesame oil
1 tablespoon gluten-free tamari
Dash cayenne pepper

Combine all ingredients in a bowl and mix with a fork.

Add water in 1-tablespoon increments to reach desired consistency.

Free of
casein, corn, dairy, eggs, fish, gluten

Prep time
5 minutes

Total time
5 minutes

Makes about
2 cups (48 1-teaspoon servings)

Per Teaspoon
Calories: 5
Calories from fat: 4
Total fat: 0.5 g
Saturated fat: 0 g
Cholesterol: 0 mg
Sodium: 6 mg
Carbohydrates: 0 g
Fiber: 0 g
Sugars: 0 g
Protein: 0 g
Vitamin A: 0% DV
Vitamin C: 9% DV
Calcium: 2% DV
Iron: 3% DV

Enriching Eggless Mayo

This recipe is from my friend Dr. Elizabeth Kirkland, who has many different food intolerances and must mind what she eats. After realizing that eggs were something she should omit from her diet, she came up with this fantastic egg-free recipe. Use it as you would regular mayonnaise.

1½ tablespoons quinoa flour
½ teaspoon salt
¼ teaspoon dry mustard
1 cup cold water
½ cup extra virgin olive oil
1 tablespoon apple cider vinegar
Pinch of paprika
Salt and pepper to taste

Combine flour, salt, mustard, and ¼ cup of the water in a mixing bowl and stir well. Put the remaining water in a saucepan and bring to a boil. Reduce to a simmer and add the flour mixture. Stir until the mixture thickens. Cool to lukewarm.

Combine the oil and vinegar and slowly add to the mixture slowly, beating constantly. Add paprika, salt, and pepper.

The mayo will keep for a couple of weeks if refrigerated in a covered container.

Free of
casein, corn, dairy, eggs, fish, gluten, nuts

Prep time
5 minutes

Total time
15 minutes

Makes about
2 cups (96 1-tablespoon servings)

Per Serving
Calories: 12
Calories from fat: 11
Total fat: 1 g
Saturated fat: 0 g
Cholesterol: 0 mg
Sodium: 0 mg
Carbohydrates: 0 g
Fiber: 0 g
Sugars: 0 g
Protein: 0 g
Vitamin A: 0% DV
Vitamin C: 0% DV
Calcium: 0% DV
Iron: 1% DV

Notes

Chapter 1

1. J. M. Hwang and M. G. Varma, "Surgery for Inflammatory Bowel Disease," *World Journal of Gastroenterology* 14, no. 17 (2008): 2678–90, http://www.ncbi.nlm.nih.gov/pmc/articles/PMC2709047 (accessed January 23, 2012).
2. O. Bernell, A. Lapidus, and G. Hellers, "Risk Factors for Surgery and Postoperative Reccurance in Crohn's Disease," *Annals of Surgery* 231, no. 1 (2000): 38–45, http://www.ncbi.nlm.nih.gov/pmc/articles /PMC1420963 (accessed January 23, 2012).
3. R. S. Sandler et al., "The Burden of Selected Digestive Diseases in the United States," *Gastroenterology* 122, no. 5 (2002): 1500–1511, http://www.ncbi.nlm.nih.gov/pubmed/11984534 (accessed January 23, 2012).
4. Ibid.
5. Crohn's and Colitis Foundation of America, "About Crohn's Disease," 2009, http://www.ccfa.org/info/about/crohns (accessed November 8, 2011).
6. U. Volta et al., "High Prevalence of Celiac Disease in Italian General Population," *Digestive Diseases and Sciences* 46, no. 7 (2001): 1500–1505, http://www.ncbi.nlm.nih.gov/pubmed/11478502 (accessed January 23, 2012).
7. W. A. Rowe, "Inflammatory Bowel Disease—Epidemiology," http://emedicine.medscape.com/article/179037-overview#a0156 (accessed November 8, 2011).
8. C. M. Bernstein, "2010—The Year of Inflammatory Bowel Disease: A Special Interview with WDHD Campaign Leader, Dr. Charles Bernstein," *Journal of Clinical Gastroenterology* 44, no. 8 (2010): v–vi.

9. Centers for Disease Control and Prevention, "Inflammatory Bowel Disease (IBD)," http://www.cdc.gov/ibd (accessed April 23, 2012).

10. R. Pullan et al., "Transdermal Nicotine for Active Ulcerative Colitis," *New England Journal of Medicine* 330 (1994): 811–15, http://www.nejm.org/doi/full/10.1056/NEJM199403243301202 (accessed January 23, 2012).

11. J. Wolf, ed., "Inflammatory Bowel Disease Fact Sheet," http://www.womenshealth.gov/publications/our-publications/fact-sheet/inflammatory-bowel-disease.cfm#b (accessed January 23, 2012).

12. The University of Utah Genetic Science Learning Center, "What Is Epigenetics?" http://learn.genetics.utah.edu/content/epigenetics (accessed April 14, 2012).

13. K. R. Gardiner, "Operative Management of Small Bowel Crohn's Disease," *Surgical Clinics of North America* 87, no. 3 (2007): 587–610, http://www.ncbi.nlm.nih.gov/pubmed/17560414 (accessed January 23, 2012).

14. Ibid.

15. *Supersize Me*, DVD, directed by Morgan Spurlock (Samuel Goldwyn Films, 2004).

16. W. Bumgardner, "How Many Pedometer Steps per Day Are Enough?" http://walking.about.com/cs/measure/a/locke122004.htm (accessed January 23, 2012).

17. P. Levine, *In an Unspoken Voice: How the Body Releases Trauma and Restores Goodness*, (Berkeley, CA: North Atlantic Books, 2010), 120–25; http://tinyurl.com/cluhdxp (accessed July 19, 2012).

18. F. Orrego and C. Quintana, "Darwin's Illness: A Final Diagnosis," *Notes & Records of the Royal Society* 61, no. 1 (2007): 23–29; http://rsnr.royalsocietypublishing.org/content/61/1/23.full (accessed July 19, 2012).

19. C. Darwin, *The Expression of the Emotions in Man and Animals* (London: John Murray, 1872), 69.

20. World Health Organization, "World Health Organization Assesses the World's Health Systems," http://www.who.int/inf-pr-2000/en/pr2000-44.html (accessed January 23, 2012).

21. "Blue Zones," interview with Mehmet Oz, by Oprah Winfrey, *The Oprah Winfrey Show*, 2010.

22. G. Null et al., "Death by Medicine," *Life Extension*, 2003, http://www.lef.org/magazine/mag2004/mar2004_awsi_death_01.htm (accessed January 23, 2012).

Chapter 2

1. R. Melillo, *Disconnected Kids* (New York: Perigree, 2009), 43.
2. P. J. D'Adamo, *Eat Right 4 Your Type* (New York: Putnam Adult, 1996), 52.
3. D. Royall et al., "Comparison of Amino Acid v Peptide Based Enteral Diets in Active Crohn's Disease: Clinical and Nutritional Outcome," *GUT* 35, no. 6 (1994): 783–87, http://www.ncbi.nlm.nih.gov/pmc /articles/PMC1374879 (accessed January 23, 2012).
4. S. Bentz, "Clinical Relevance of IgG Antibodies Against Food Antigens in Crohn's Disease: A Double-Blind Cross-Over Diet Intervention Study," *Digestion* 81, no. 4 (2010): 252–64, http://www.ncbi.nlm .nih.gov/pubmed/20130407 (accessed January 23, 2012).
5. E. M. Workman et al., "Diet in the Management of Crohn's Disease," *Human Nutrition: Applied Nutrition* 38, no. 6 (1984): 469–73, http:// www.ncbi.nlm.nih.gov/pubmed/6526690 (accessed January 23, 2012).
6. A. Emmanuel, "IgG and Gastroentestinal Disorders—2007," http:// www.foodsmatter.com/allergy_intolerance/miscellaneous/articles /igg_emmanuel.html (accessed January 23, 2012).

Chapter 3

1. B. A. Pribila et al., "Improved Lactose Digestion and Tolerance among African-American Adolescent Girls Fed a Dairy-Rich Diet," *Journal of the American Dietetic Association* 100, no. 5 (2000): 524–28, http://www.ncbi.nlm.nih.gov/pubmed/10812376 (accessed January 23, 2012).
2. I. Abubakar et al., "A Case-Control Study of Drinking Water and Dairy Products in Crohn's Disease—Further Investigation of the Possible Role of Mycobacterium Avium Paratuberculosis," *American Journal of Epidemiology* 165, no. 7 (2007): 776–83.
3. M. Nestle, *Food Politics: How the Food Industry Influences Nutrition and Health* (Berkeley: University of California Press, 2007), 104.
4. Ibid., 81.
5. U. S. Census Bureau, "Internet Users Stats in 2009 for the Americas," 2009, http://www.census.gov/hhes/computer/publications/2009 .html (accessed July 25, 2012).
6. *King Korn*, DVD, directed by Aaron Woolf (Balcony Releasing Films, 2008).

7. J. S. de Vendômois et al., "A Comparison of the Effects of Three GM Corn Varieties on Mammalian Health," *International Journal of Biological Sciences* 5, no. 7 (2009): 706–26.

8. J. Rosenthal, *Integrative Nutrition* (New York: Integrative Nutrition Publishing, 2008), 9.

9. U. S. Geological Survey, "Pesticides in the Nation's Streams and Ground Water, 1992–2001—A Summary," 2006, http://pubs.water .usgs.gov/fs20063028 (accessed 29 November 2011).

10. Rosenthal, *Integrative Nutrition*, 9.

11. J. Rubin, *Patient Heal Thyself* (Evanston, IL: Freedom Press, 2003), 9.

12. Rosenthal, *Integrative Nutrition*, 9.

13. C. Benbrook, D. R. Davis, and P. K. Andrews, "Organic Center Response to the FSA Study," Boulder, CO: The Organic Center, 2009, http://www.organic-center.org/science.nutri.php?action=view &report_id=157 (accessed July 25, 2012); C. Benbrook et al., "New Evidence Confirms the Nutritional Superiority of Plant-Based Organic Foods," The Organic Center, 2008, http://www.organic-center .org/science.nutri.php?action=view&report_id=126 (accessed July 25, 2012); F. E. Bear, S. J. Toth, and A. L. Prince. "Variation in Mineral Composition of Vegetables," *Soil Science Society American Proceedings*, 13(1948):380–84.

14. J. F. Mayberry and J. Rhodes, "Epidemiological Aspects of Crohn's Disease: A Review of the Literature," *Gut* 25, no. 8 (1984): 886–99, http://www.ncbi.nlm.nih.gov/pmc/articles/PMC1432571 (accessed January 25, 2012).

15. N. Appleton, *Lick the Sugar Habit*, 2nd ed. (New York: Avery, 1996), 60.

16. E. Gottschall, *Breaking the Vicious Cycle: Intestinal Health Through Diet*, rev. ed., (Baltimore, MD: Kirkton Press, 1994), 27.

17. Gottschall, *Breaking the Vicious Cycle*, 12.

18. Rosenthal, *Integrative Nutrition*, 9.

19. Appleton, *Lick the Sugar Habit*, 82

20. Rosenthal, *Integrative Nutrition*, 9.

21. A. L. Gittleman, *Get the Sugar Out* (New York: Three Rivers Press, 1996), 44.

22. S. Braun, *Buzz: The Science and Lore of Alcohol and Caffeine* (New York: Oxford University Press, 1996), 56.

23. E. Strain et al., "Caffeine Dependence Syndrome," *Journal of the American Medical Association* 272, no. 13 (1994): 1043–1048.

24. D. Robertson et al., "Effect of Caffeine on Plasma Renin Activity, Catecholamines and Blood Pressure," *New England Journal of Medicine* 298, no. 4 (1978): 181–86, http://www.ncbi.nlm.nih.gov/pubmed /339084 (accessed January 26, 2012).

25. S. R. Brown, P. A. Cann, and N. W. Read, "Effects of Coffee on Distal Colon Function," *GUT International Journal of Gastroenterology and Hepatology* 31, no. 4 (1990): 450–53, http://www.ncbi.nlm.nih.gov /pmc/articles/PMC1378422 (accessed January 26, 2012).

26. D. J. Roca, G. D. Schiller, and D. H. Farb, "Chronic Caffeine or Theophylline Exposure Reduces Gamma-Aminobutyric Acid/Benzodiazepine Receptor Site Interactions," *Molecular Pharmacology* 33, no. 5 (1988): 481–85, http://www.ncbi.nlm.nih.gov/pubmed/2835648 (accessed January 26, 2012).

27. S. Cohen and G. H. Booth, Jr., "Gastric acid secretion and Lower-Esophageal-Sphincter Pressure in Response to Coffee and Caffeine," *New England Journal of Medicine* 293, no. 18 (1975): 897–99, http:// www.ncbi.nlm.nih.gov/pubmed/1177987 (accessed January 26, 2012).

28. R. Utley, "Nutritional Factors Associated with Wound Healing in the Elderly," *Ostomy Wound Management* 38, no. 3 (1992): 22, 24, 26–27, http://www.ncbi.nlm.nih.gov/pubmed/1580969 (accessed January 26, 2012).

Chapter 4

1. Jordan S. Rubin and Gary Gordon, *Patient Heal Thyself: A Remarkable Health Program Combining Ancient Wisdom with Groundbreaking Clinical Research* (Topanga, CA: Freedom Press, 2004), 20.

2. Joshua Rosenthal, *Integrative Nutrition* (New York: Integrative Nutrition Publishing, 2008), 9.

3. David Peters and Kenneth R. Pelletier, *New Medicine: Complete Family Health Guide* (New York: DK Publishing, 2007), 216.

4. Rosenthal, *Integrative Nutrition*, 9.

5. Mary G. Enig, "Coconut: In Support of Good Health in the 21st Century" (2001). http://articles.mercola.com/sites/articles/archive /2001/07/28/coconut-health.aspx (accessed April 16, 2012).

6. Paul Pitchford, *Healing with Whole Foods: Asian Traditions and Modern Nutrition* (Berkeley, CA: North Atlantic Books, 2002), 542.

7. Ibid., 622.

8. Ibid., 621.

9. Rubin and Gordon, *Patient Heal Thyself*, 256.

10. Pitchford, *Healing with Whole Foods*, 537.

11. Ibid., 539.

12. Rosenthal, *Integrative Nutrition*, 9.

13. A. Belluzi et al., "Effects of New Fish Oil Derivative on Fatty Acid Phospholipid-Membrane Pattern in a Group of Crohn's Disease Patients," *Digestive Disease Science* 39, no. 12 (1994): 2589–94, http://www.ncbi.nlm.nih.gov/pubmed/7995183 (accessed January 26, 2012).

14. Patrick Holford, *The New Optimum Nutrition Bible* (Berkeley, CA: Crossing Press, 2004), 394.

Chapter 5

1. Jordan S. Rubin, *The Maker's Diet* (Lake Mary, FL: Siloam, 2004), 64.

2. R. R. Watson and T. K. Leonard, "Selenium and Vitamins A, C and E: Nutrients with Cancer Prevention Properties," *Journal of the American Dietetic Association* 86, no. 4 (1986): 505–510, http://www.ncbi.nlm.nih.gov/pubmed/3514733 (accessed on January 26, 2012).

3. C. D. Gillen et al., "Ulcerative Colitis and Crohn's Disease: A Comparison of the Colorectal Cancer Risk in Extensive Colitis," *GUT International Journal of Gastroenterology and Hepatology* 35, no. 11 (1994): 1590–92, http://www.ncbi.nlm.nih.gov/pmc/articles/PMC 1375617 (accessed January 26, 2012).

4. Rubin, *The Maker's Diet*, 10.

5. Ibid., 28.

6. Ibid., 200.

7. Patrick Holford, *The New Optimum Nutrition Bible* (Berkeley, CA: Crossing Press, 2004), 157.

8. T. S. King, M. Elia, and J. O. Hunter, "Abnormal Colonic Fermentation in Irritable Bowel Syndrome," *Lancet* 352, no. 9135:1187–89, http://www.ncbi.nlm.nih.gov/pubmed/9777836 (accessed January 26, 2012).

9. Holford, *The New Optimum Nutrition Bible*, 190.

10. Holford, *The New Optimum Nutrition Bible*, 228.

11. Paul Pitchford, *Healing with Whole Foods: Asian Traditions and Modern Nutrition* (Berkeley, CA: North Atlantic Books, 2002), 210.

12. K. Kenigsburg et al., "Use of Charcoal for Treating Inflammatory Conditions," in *Newsday*, ed. Jamie Talan (January 2006), http://www.listen2yourgut.com/charcoal.php (accessed January 26, 2012).

13. Holford, *The New Optimum Nutrition Bible*, 228.
14. Holford, *The New Optimum Nutrition Bible*, 229.
15. T. E. Towheed et al., "Glucosamine Therapy for Treating Osteoarthritis," Cochrane Database of Systemic Reviews 2, no. CD002946 (2005), http://www.ncbi.nlm.nih.gov/pubmed/15846645 (accessed on January 26, 2012).

Chapter 6

1. P. J. D'Adamo, *Eat Right 4 Your Type* (New York: Putnam Adult, 1996), 67.

Chapter 7

1. Joseph Mercola, "Help Your Heart: 71% of Those Who Drank This Lowered Their Blood Pressure" (2011), http://articles.mercola.com/sites/articles/archive/2011/11/27/coconut-water-ultimate-rehydrator.aspx (accessed June 26, 2012).

Resources

Metametrix Clinical Laboratory
(800) 221-4640   www.metametrix.com
This lab offers a Triad Profile—blood/urine is used to test food intolerances, allergies, and organic acid profiles from which individualized vitamin/mineral/amino-acid formulas may be ordered. This testing is highly recommended for those with IBD.

Enterolabs
(972) 686-6869   www.enterolab.com
This lab offers accurate DNA testing for gluten, casein intolerance, and sensitivities. Testing is highly recommended for those with suspected food intolerances who have not been diagnosed by any other means.

Metabolic Maintenance Products
(800) 772-7873   www.metabolicmaintenance.com
This company provides individualized vitamin, mineral, and amino-acid formulas based upon Metametrix Triad Profiles.

If you can find a nutritionist or physician who works with Metabolic Maintenance (MM), you will be able to order customized vitamins and minerals that are appropriate for your own unique IBD needs. Please contact MM for assistance in locating a practitioner who works with this company.

Once the MM clinician and your nutritional consultant have completed your individualized formula, a representative from Metabolic Maintenance will contact you to arrange delivery of supplementation.

The individualized amino-acid formula can be purchased in capsules or powder form. You can administer the powder by whatever means necessary (i.e., in applesauce, juices, smoothies, or sauces), or you may choose to encapsulate the powder yourself (see Wonder Laboratories, below).

IMPORTANT: The dosage on the bottle represents what would be appropriate for an adult. Children under twelve should have approximately half the dosage, but it is important to be case specific and consult with a doctor before administering any treatments.

The Garden of Life
(866) 465-0051   www.gardenoflife.com
Garden of Life offers a number of products recommended in this book for IBD. Its most popular products for digestion are:
- Primal Defense (HSO probiotic)
- FYI Restore (contains bromelain to control intestinal information)
- Omega-Zyme (high-quality digestive enzyme)
- whole-food multivitamins
- RAW ONE multivitamins

To boost energy levels, Garden of Life offers a product called Clear Energy (whole-food B-vitamin complex).

Nordic Naturals
(800) 662-2544   www.nordicnaturals.com
This company offers the highest-quality fish-oil supplement, with special formulas geared toward children and adults. It is highly recommended for intestinal inflammation. Several varieties are available:
- Arctic Cod Liver Oil 8 oz. (strawberry, orange)
- Pro Omega 90 Soft Gels (chewable)
- Pro Omega 60/120 caps (lemon)
- Omega 3-6-9 Junior Liquid (lemon flavored)

Coromega Company
(877) 275-3725   www.coromegakids.com
This company offers omega-3 fish oil that is palatable to children and picky adults. This formula is gluten free but contains egg yolks.

Mega Foods
(800) 848-2542   www.metagenics.com   www.megafood.com
This company offers an array of quality supplements, including basic vitamin/mineral formulation, probiotics, digestive enzymes, and herbal and homeopathic remedies.

Recommended products include the following:
- Ultra Flora PlusDF (powdered and encapsulated probiotics)
- Ultracare for Kids (and Adults)—A high-quality nutritional medical food that contains a low-allergy-potential rice-protein base suitable for those with dairy, gluten, or soy sensitivities. It is an excellent source of dairy-free calcium, prebiotic fructooligosaccharides (carbohydrates that many feel should become a greater portion of the diet as they support a healthy digestive tract), and essential fatty acids.
- Ultra Potent-C 1000 (90 tablets)—A good vitamin-C supplement that can be used in specific cases when increased antioxidants are needed.

Transformation Enzyme Products
(800) 777-1474   www.transformationenzymes.com
This company offers quality digestive enzymes.
    I recommend Digestzyme—powdered and encapsulated.

Boiron Homeopathic Products
(610) 325-7464   www.boiron.com
Offering quality homeopathics for digestion. Here are my favorites to recommend:
- Acidil—excellent for indigestion
- Antimonium crudum—use for indigestion with nausea
- Arsenicum album—perfect for trips when you are flaring-up or have traveler's diarrhea
- Carbo vegetabilis—aids abdominal bloating and gas
- Chelidonium majus—aids indigestion and nausea

Hylands/Standard Homeopathics
(800) 624-9659   www.hylands.com
- Calm Forte is used for anxiety and/or sleep difficulties.
- Hyland's Hemmorex Ointment is for palliative relief from the misery and discomfort of simple piles or hemorrhoids.
- Hyland's Diarrex is for all-natural relief from the not-so-pleasant effects of diarrhea.
- Hyland's Gas provides natural relief of symptoms of flatulence, belching, and gas due to improper digestion or gastric upset.

- Hyland's Motion Sickness provides natural relief for nausea and dizziness associated with, or aggravated by, motion.
- Hyland's Indigestion is a traditional homeopathic formula for the relief of symptoms of dyspepsia and upset stomach due to hyperacidity or improper diet.
- Hyland's Upset Stomach provides natural relief of symptoms of flatulence, belching, and gas due to improper digestion or gastric upset.

Always use caution with homeopathics if you are on any medication. Generally, these are very safe products, but always do your homework.

Wonder Laboratories

(800) 992-1672   www.wonderlabs.com

This company supplies empty gelatin capsules with a capsule-filling machine (at very cost-effective rates) for use with individualized vitamin/mineral formulas from Metabolic Maintenance. Many find it much easier to fill capsules with powdered formula themselves, as individualized formulas are not available in capsules (they come in powder only). Some patients have difficulty with the taste of the powder. Therefore, the option of filling capsules at home is best, if you can tolerate swallowing them.

Index

Boldface page numbers refer to recipes located in the text.

A

adenosine triphosphate (ATP), 21, 47
agave, 92–93
ALA. *See* alpha-linolenic acid
ALCAT (test lab), 56
allergic reactions, 41–43. *See also* food
  allergies
allicin, 124
Allie's Applesauce Bread, **151**
Almond Butter and Jelly Breakfast
  Pizza, **154**
Almond Millet Pilaf, **213**
almonds: Almond Butter and Jelly
  Breakfast Pizza, **154**; Almond Millet
  Pilaf, **213**; Cheery Cherry Almond
  Cupcookie, **240–241**; "Coco-nutty"
  Almond Pancakes, **149**; Homemade
  Vanilla Almond Milk, **168**
alpha-linolenic acid (ALA), 123
American diet, 82, 84, 97, 102
American Dietetic Association, 118
American Journal of Epidemiology, 84
American lifestyle, 19–22
amino acids: essential, 107, 110; glutathione, 37; therapy, 47, 101
amylase, 122, 139
anaphylactic shock, 42
antibiotics: bacteria and, 25, 119–120;
  probiotics *vs.*, 119–120
antibodies, 39–40, 120
antigens, 39
anti-inflammatory diet menu, 111–112
anti-inflammatory food pyramid, 102
anti-inflammatory foods, 100, 101–102

anti-inflammatory lunch ideas, 113–114
antioxidants: astaxanthin, 145; oxidative
  stress and, 118; in tea, 99
appetizers and snacks, 102, 175–182
Apple Cinnamon Granola, **181**
Apple Rosemary Cornish Game Hens,
  194–195
apples: Apple Cinnamon Granola, **181**;
  Apple Rosemary Cornish Game
  Hens, **194–195**
asparagus: Grilled Asparagus, Rice, and
  Peas, **220**
astaxanthin, 145
asthma, 41
Atkins, Robert, 109
Atkins Diet, 109
ATP. *See* adenosine triphosphate
Authentic and Easy Fried Rice, **209**
autoimmune response, 39
avocado: Kiwi Avocado Salad, **231**;
  Simply Simple Avocado Dip, **251**

B

baby food, 105, 163
bacteria: antibiotics and, 25, 119–120;
  *Mycobacterium avium paratubercu-
  losis*, 84; probiotics and, 37, 82, 119–120.
  See also homeostatic soil organisms
Baked Coconut Shrimp, **205**
Banana Cherry Fruit Squares, **242**
bananas: Banana Cherry Fruit Squares,
  242; Buttery Banana Cupcakes, **180**;
  Carob Chip Banana Pancakes, **148**;
  Frozen Dark Chocolate Banana Pops,

247; Mighty Mango Banana Cream Machine, **244**; Pecan 'n' Banana Breakfast Bread, **155**

Band-Aid approach, 24–25

beans, 187–190; Creamy Coconut Adzuki Beans, **188**; Mexican Fiesta Rice 'n' Beans with Veggies, **190**; Tomato Simmered String Beans, **226**

beef, 191; Slow Cook Beef Tender, **201**

Bernard, Claude, 20

Bernstein, Charles, 14

beverages, 163–174. *See also specific beverages*

biodiversity, 89

Blissful Breakfast Wrap, **160**

blood sugar, 92

blood testing, 49, 58–63, 83

The Blood Type Diet (D'Adamo), 46

blood-type diet, 46, 129, 130–135

blue zones, 23–24, 108

Blueberry Walnut Waffles, Wonderful, **156**

The Blue Zones: Lessons for Living Longer from the People Who've Lived the Longest (Buettner), 23

Boiron Homeopathic Products, 265

boswellia, 127–128

bowel movements, 51, 82, 109; caffeine and, 97–98; urgency, 115–116

BRAT (bananas, rice, apples, and toast), 106

bread: Allie's Applesauce Bread, **151**; Pecan 'n' Banana Breakfast Bread, **155**

breakfast recipes, 146–162

Broccoli, Roasted Lemon, **217**

bromelain, 38, 101, 105, 122

brown rice, 106; Authentic and Easy Fried Rice, **209**; Brown Rice Pudding, **245**; Brown Rice Quesadillas, **179**; Mexican Fiesta Rice 'n' Beans with Veggies, **190**; Sesame Glazed Ginger Tuna Steaks with Brown Rice, **207**; Very Vanilla Rice Milk, **170**

Brown Rice Pudding, **245**

Brown Rice Quesadillas, **179**

buckwheat, 106–107; Good Morning Buckwheat, **161**

Buettner, Dan, 23

butter, substitutions for, 74

Buttery Banana Cupcakes, **180**

C

cabbage, 105–106

caffeine, 97–99; reducing or eliminating, 96; withdrawal, 97, 99

calcium, 75, 84

cancer, 118

candida, 110–111

Caramel Balls, Nutty Natural, **233**

carbohydrates: complex, 92; refined, 86, 92

Carob Chip Banana Pancakes, **148**

Carrot and Raisin Salad, **227**

carrots: Carrot and Raisin Salad, **227**; Roasted Carrots with Molasses and Dill, **222**

casein, 45, 46, 138

Cashew Rice Noodles, **211**

casomorphin, 45

Cauliflower, Roasted, and White Wine Pasta, **214**

CDC. *See* Centers for Disease Control and Prevention

celery, 106

celiac disease: causes of, 11, 13, 15; symptoms of, 11, 13, 100; treatment for, 11–12, 100–101

Centers for Disease Control and Prevention (CDC), 12

charcoal, 125–126

Cheerfully Cherry Pecan Salad, **229**

Cheery Cherry Almond Cupcookie, **240–241**

cheese, substitutions for, 74

cherries: Banana Cherry Fruit Squares, **242**; Cheerfully Cherry Pecan Salad, **229**; Cheery Cherry Almond Cupcookie, **240–241**; Pineapple Cherrylicious Explosion, **174**

chewing food, 139–140

chicken: Chicken and Veggie Tacos, **193**; Grilled Chicken and Shiitake Mushrooms with Polenta, **192**; Mom's Classic Chicken Soup, **184**; Oven-Roasted Chicken and Potatoes, **200**; Simple Grilled Chicken, **191**; Simply

Classic Lemon Pepper Rosemary Chicken, **202**
Chicken and Veggie Tacos, **193**
Chocolate Banana Pops, Frozen Dark, **247**
chopsticks, children's, 139–140
Christie's Groovy Green Machine Juice, **169**
Clean Fifteen list, 144–145, 168
"Clinical Relevance of IgG Antibodies Against Food Antigens in Crohn's Disease: A Double-Blind Cross-Over Intervention Study," 51
coconut: Baked Coconut Shrimp, **205**; Creamy Coconut Adzuki Beans, **188**
coconut milk, 101, 104, 167
coconut oil, 104, 107
coconut water, 104, 163; Coconut Water Coolada, **165**
Coconut Water Coolada, **165**
"Coco-nutty" Almond Pancakes, **149**
coffee, 97–99
colitis: causes and symptoms of, 12–13, 81–82, 143; treatment for, 81–83, 143–144
Collard Green Stuffing, Sweet, **219**
Comfort Cranberry Sauce, **253**
community farms, 145
congee (slow-cooked grain), 144
corn: genetically modified, 87–88; substitutes and avoiding, 72; as top allergen, 46
Cornish Game Hens, Apple Rosemary, **194–195**
Coromega Company, 264
COX-1 and COX-2 enzymes, 128
cranberries: Comfort Cranberry Sauce, **253**; Cranberry Strawberry Breakfast Bars, **157**; Strawberry Cranberry Smoothie, **164**
Cranberry Strawberry Breakfast Bars, **157**
Creamy Coconut Adzuki Beans, **188**
Creamy Peanut Sauce, **254**
Crohn's and Colitis Foundation of America, 13
Crohn's disease: causes of, 12, 24, 37, 84, 90–91; symptoms of, 1–3, 12, 37, 130;
tests for, 1, 4; treatments for, 1–5, 26, 37–38, 129–130
crowding-out theory, 138
curcumin, 127
Curry Turkey Tenders, **197**
cytokines, 14, 40, 43

D

D'Adamo, Peter, 46, 130
Daily Value (DV), 144
dairy: alternatives for, 38; intolerances, 1–2, 37, 138; organic products, 87; in rotation diet, 69; substitutes and avoiding, 74–75, 121, 163; as top allergen, 46; USDA guidelines for, 84, 86
Dairy-Free Whipped Rice Cream, **243**
Daphne's story, 115–116
Darwin, Charles, 20
Dean, Carolyn, 25
"Death by Medicine" (Null, Dean, Feldman, Rasio, and Smith), 25
dehydration, 91, 104, 163, 170
Department of Health and Human Services, U.S., 14
desserts. *See* snacks and desserts
DHA. *See* docosahexaenoic acid
diet: American diet, 82, 84, 97, 102; anti-inflammatory diet menu, 111–112; Atkins Diet, 109; blood-type diet, 46, 129, 130–135; food-elimination diet, 10, 48–49, 63–65; gluten-free diet, 4, 11; low-fat diet, 47, 123; reintroduction diet, 65–68; rotation diet, 49, 59, 69–71; vegetarian and vegan diet, 108–111; wellness through dietary change, ix–x, 4–6
Digestion, 51
digestion diary, 32, 57–58
digestion quiz, 29–33
digestive enzymes, 10, 139, 265
digestive system, 44–45
dips. *See* dressings, sauces, and dips
Dirty Dozen list, 144, 168, 169
Division of Gastroenterology (Toronto, Canada), 47
docosahexaenoic acid (DHA), 123–124
dressings, sauces, and dips, 216, 248–255
drugs. *See* medications
DV. *See* Daily Value

E

Eastern medicine, 15

eatwellguide.org, 145

edema, 39

eggplant: Sun-Dried Tomato Grilled Eggplant, **224**; Zesty Zucchini or Eggplant Sticks, **238–239**

eggs: Groovy Green Eggs and Ham, **159**; intolerance to, **37**; organic, 145; Poached Eggs with Honey Mustard Spinach, **152**; Pumpkin Pie Healthy Egg Cream, **172**; substitutes and avoiding, 76, 233; as top allergen, 46

eicosapentaenoic acid (EPA), 123–124

Ellis, Curt, 87

Emmanuel, Anton, 51–52

emotions, 20–21; emotional balance, 67; emotional symptoms of food intolerances, 67–68

Enriching Eggless Mayo, **255**

Enterolabs, 263

Environmental Working Group (EWG), 144–145, 168, 169

enzymes, 121–123; how to take, 123; types of, 10, 38, 122–123, 128, 139, 265

EPA. *See* eicosapentaenoic acid

epigenetics, 15

Erick's story, 143–144

essential amino acids, 107, 110

essential fatty acids, 107–108

EWG. *See* Environmental Working Group

exercise, 11, 19

The Expression of the Emotions in Man and Animals (Darwin), 20

extrinsic factor, 108, 125

F

Falafel Nuggets with Tomato Sauce, **176–177**

Far-Out Fruit Salad, **228**

Feldman, Martin, 25

Fellas, Penny, 176

fish and seafood, 203–207; wild-caught compared to farm-raised, 145, 203. *See also specific fish and seafood*

fish oil, 124, 264

flare-ups: beverages for, 163–164, 169, 171, 173; enzymes for, 122; food aver-

sions and, 38; fruit and vegetables for, 103–106; soups for, 183; vitamin C for, 126

flavor of organic foods, 89

flushable wipes, 8

food addiction: coffee, 97–99; food intolerances and, 37, 44–45; sugar, 91–93, 100–101

food allergies: food intolerances *versus*, x, 5, 41–43; sample allergen-free menu, 135–136; substitutes and avoiding eight allergens, 71–80; top eight allergens, 46, 84–85. *See also* IgE reactions

food aversions, 38, 82

food diary, 31–32, 48, 56–57, 103, 138

food enzymes, 122

food industry, 85

food intolerances, 36–80; case study, 52–56; causes of, 139; food addiction and, 37, 44–45; food allergies *versus*, x, 5, 41–43; identifying, 38–39; impacts of, 36–37; physical and emotional symptoms of, 67–68; proteins and, 4, 45, 46–47; quiz, 47–50; science behind, 50–56; tests for, 10, 32, 37, 47–50, 52–56. *See also specific foods*

Food Matters (Emmanuel), 51–52

food politics, 83–86

food pyramids: anti-inflammatory, 102; USDA, 85–86

food sensitivities: common, 46; concurrent, 11; recurrence of, 69. *See also* food intolerances

food-elimination diet, 10, 48–49, 63–65; planning for, 65; withdrawal symptoms with, 64

France, 21

Frank's story, 37–38, 45

Frozen Dark Chocolate Banana Pops, **247**

fruit, 102–106; eating more, 91–92; Far-Out Fruit Salad, **228**; for flare-ups, 103–106; puréed, 104–105. *See also specific fruit*

Functional Disconnection Syndrome, 44

G

GABA (gamma-aminobutyric acid), 98

Garden of Life, 264

garlic, 124; Roasted Garlic Hummus, **189**

genetics, *ix*; genetic testing, 4; genetically modified foods, 87–88. *See also* epigenetics

Genova Diagnostics, 56

Gentle Ginger Peppermint Chiller, **173**

ginger, 128; Gentle Ginger Peppermint Chiller, **173**; Grilled Salmon with Honey Ginger Sauce, **204**; Sesame Glazed Ginger Tuna Steaks with Brown Rice, **207**

gliadin, 13

glutathione, 37

gluten, 4; as common sensitivity, 46; sources of, 13, 45, 78; substitutes and avoiding, 77–78

gluten intolerance, 4

gluten-free diet, 4, 11

gluten-free grains, 107, 208

glutomorphin, 45

goals, 18, 33–34

Good Morning Buckwheat, **161**

Gottschall, Elaine, 36

grains: avoiding, 36, 78; congee, 144; gluten-free, 107, 208; as not part of human diet, 46; whole grains, 92, 106–107. *See also specific grains*

granola: Apple Cinnamon Granola, **181**; Granola and Yogurt Parfait, **153**

Granola and Yogurt Parfait, **153**

Grilled Asparagus, Rice, and Peas, **220**

Grilled Chicken and Shiitake Mushrooms with Polenta, **192**

Grilled Halibut Steaks with Mustard, **203**

Grilled Peaches, **178**

Grilled Salmon with Honey Ginger Sauce, **204**

grocery shopping cards, 71–80

Groovy Green Eggs and Ham, **159**

H

Halibut Steaks with Mustard, Grilled, **203**

Ham, Groovy Green Eggs and, **159**

Hannan, Nuri, 254

happiness, 19

Healthnotes, 118

Hermon-Taylor, Jon, 84

Holford, Patrick, 128

holistic approach, 5–6; American lifestyle and, 19–22; to positive lifestyle changes, *x*, 28–29; reasons for, 17–18; standard medical approach compared to, 5, 9

holistic nutrition, 83

Homemade Vanilla Almond Milk, **168**

homeostatic soil organisms (HSOs), 89, 119, 121

honey: Grilled Salmon with Honey Ginger Sauce, **204**; Poached Eggs with Honey Mustard Spinach, **152**

hormones, 20–21, 55; stress hormones, 45, 97

HSOs. *See* homeostatic soil organisms

Human Nutrition: Applied Nutrition, 51

Hummus, Roasted Garlic, **189**

humor, 7–8, 19, 140–141

hydrochloric acid, 125

Hylands/Standard Homeopathics, 265–266

hypersensitivity: delayed hypersensitivity and IgG, 43; immediate hypersensitivity and IgE, 42–43

I

IBD. *See* inflammatory bowel disease

IBS. *See* irritable bowel syndrome

ibuprofen, 128

ice cream, substitutions for, 74

ice pops, 171, 236

IgA (immunoglobulin), 40

IgD (immunoglobulin), 40

IgE (immunoglobulin), 40

IgE reactions (food allergies), 42–43

IgG (immunoglobulin), 40

IgG Food Antibody Blood Test, 58–63

IgG reactions (food intolerances), 42–43

IgM (immunoglobulin), 40

ileoanal pouch anal anastomosis, 17

ileostomy, 16–17

immune system, 14; boosts to, 120, 126; environmental factors affecting, 41; parts of body attacked by, 41; understanding, 39–43

immunoglobulins, 40

In an Unspoken Voice: How the Body

Releases Trauma and Restores Goodness (Levine), 20
indigenous enzymes, 122
inflammation: causes of, 101; healing, 5; role of, 39
inflammatory bowel disease (IBD), 1; causes and symptoms of, *ix*, 7, 11–13; science behind, 14–15, 50–56; Western medicine treatment methods, 15–17; who gets IBD, 13–14
Institute for Integrative Nutrition, 17, 35
International Journal of Biological Sciences study, 87–88
intrinsic factor, 108, 124–125
invertase, 122
irradiated food, 87
irritable bowel syndrome (IBS): study, 52; symptoms and treatment for, 12, 115–116
IsoOxygene, 128
Italy, 13

J
Johne's disease, 84
Journal of Clinical Gastroenterology, 14
Journal of the American Dietetic Association, 84
juices, 105; Christie's Groovy Green Machine Juice, **169**; juice cleanse, 82

K
kasha, 106–107, 161
King Korn (documentary), 87
Kirkland, Elizabeth, 255
Kiwi Avocado Salad, **231**
Korth, Christie, *x*
Kushi, Michio, 109

L
lactase, 122
lactose intolerance, 84
leaky gut syndrome, 44–45
Lemon and Basil Quinoa, **212**
lemons: Lemon and Basil Quinoa, **212**; Roasted Lemon Broccoli, **217**; Simply Classic Lemon Pepper Rosemary Chicken, **202**
leukotrienes, 127
Levine, Peter, 20

Lichtenstein, Robert, 137
life expectancy, countries in order of, 22
lifestyle changes, *x*, 6, 17
limitations, 9–10
lipase, 122
Little Lunch Box Mini Pizzas, **210**
Loma Linda, California, 23–24, 108
low-fat diet, 47, 123
lunches, 227; anti-inflammatory lunch ideas, 113–114; Little Lunch Box Mini Pizzas, **210**

M
macrobiotics, 109
The Macrobiotic Way (Kushi), 109
magnesium absorption, 98
malabsorption, 9, 43, 47
mango: Mango-Strawberry Salad, **232**; Mighty Mango Banana Cream Machine, **244**
Mango-Strawberry Salad, **232**
MAP. *See Mycobacterium avium paratuberculosis*
Marinated Parsnips, **223**
Marvelous Maple BBQ Dressing, **250**
Mayo, Enriching Eggless, **255**
meat: intake of, 96; organic and grass-fed, 87, 145, 191. *See also* beef
medications, 2, 16; Band-Aid approach to, 24–25; common drugs and nutritional deficiencies, 26–28; risks of prescription drugs, 25–26
Mega Foods, 264–265
Melillo, Robert, 36–37, 44
menus: anti-inflammatory diet menu, 111–112; Your Menu Planner, 129, 133–135; sample allergen-free menu, 135–136
Mercola, Joseph, 91
metabolic enzymes, 122
Metabolic Maintenance Products, 263–264
metabolic profile, 26
Metametrix Clinical Laboratory, 49, 56, 58, 263
Mexican Fiesta Rice 'n' Beans with Veggies, **190**
Michael's story, 100–101
micronutrients, 47

Midwest Center for Stress and Anxiety Home program, 53
Mighty Mango Banana Cream Machine, **244**
milk, 84; substitutions for, 74
millet, 107, 110–111; Almond Millet Pilaf, **213**
mindful eating, 136–140
minerals: eating more, 89; in salt, 144
Mock Cook 'n' Serve Vanilla Pudding, **246**
molasses, 93, 222
Molecular Pharmacology, 98
Mom's Classic Chicken Soup, **184**
Mom's Mind-Blowing Stir-Fry, **198–199**
Moore, Michael, 21
motivation, 29, 140
mushrooms: Grilled Chicken and Shiitake Mushrooms with Polenta, **192**; Portobello Steaks, **225**; shiitake and maitake, **105**
mustard: Grilled Halibut Steaks with Mustard, **203**; Poached Eggs with Honey Mustard Spinach, **152**
Mycobacterium avium paratuberculosis (MAP), 84
MyPlate, USDA, 83–86

N
Naked brand smoothie drinks, 104, 169
Nana's Irresistible French Dressing, **252**
Nana's Vegetable Dip, **249**
National Academy of Sciences, 144
National Digestive Disease Information Clearing House (NDDIC), 13
National Library of Medicine, U.S., 13
natural sweeteners, 92–93, 233
nausea, 128, 165
NDDIC. *See* National Digestive Disease Information Clearing House
nervous stomach, 20
nervous system, 44–45
Nestle, Marion, 85, 86, 91
neurotransmitters, 20–21
New England Journal of Medicine, 14
New Medicine: The Complete Family Health Guide, 103
90/10 rule, 138
noodles. *See* pasta and noodles

Nordic Naturals, 264
Nourishing Potato Soup, **185**
Null, Gary, 25
nutritional counseling, *ix–x*
nutritional data, 143, 144
nutritional deficiencies, 26–28
nuts: Nutty Natural Caramel Balls, **233**; as top allergen, 46. *See also specific nuts*
Nutty Natural Caramel Balls, **233**

O
Obama, Michelle, 86
omega-3 fatty acids, 107–108, 123–124; foods with, 145, 203; how to take, 124
onions: Un-French Onion Soup, **186**; Yummy, Healthy Onion Rings, **237**
Oprah Winfrey Show, 23–24
Optimum Nutrition Bible (Holford), 128
Orange Marmalade Turkey Burgers, **196**
organic foods, 86–89; note regarding, 144–145; organic and grass-fed meat, 87, 145, 191; reasons to eat, 88–89, 169
organic gardens and farms, 86, 89, 145
Ornish, Dean, 123
Our Favorite Salmon, **206**
Oven-Roasted Chicken and Potatoes, **200**
oxidative stress, 117–118
Oz, Mehmet, 23–24

P
painkillers, nature's, 126–128
pancakes: Carob Chip Banana Pancakes, **148**; "Coco-nutty" Almond Pancakes, **149**; Sweet Potato Pancakes, **147**
pancreatic enzymes, 38
papain, 123
papaya, 105
parasympathetic nervous system (rest-and-digest system), 44
Parsnips, Marinated, **223**
pasta and noodles: Cashew Rice Noodles, **211**; Mom's Mind-Blowing Stir-Fry, **198–199**; Rice Noodles in Basil Butter Sauce, **215**; Roasted Cauliflower and White Wine Pasta, **214**; soba noodles, 106; Tomato and Pasta Salad, **208**
Patient Heal Thyself (Rubin), 3, 4

peaches: Grilled Peaches, **178**; Peachy-Keen Smoothie, **166**

Peachy-Keen Smoothie, **166**

peanuts: Creamy Peanut Sauce, **254**; substitutes and avoiding, 73; as top allergen, 46

peas, 187

Pecan 'n' Banana Breakfast Bread, **155**

pecans: Cheerfully Cherry Pecan Salad, **229**; Pecan 'n' Banana Breakfast Bread, **155**

Pepper and Potato Hash, **158**

peptidase, 123

peristalsis, 108–109, 125

pescetarians, 108

pesticides, 88, 145, 168

pH imbalance, 98

PHPPs. *See* Primary Health Puzzle Pieces

physical balance, 67

phytase, 123

pineapple, 105, 167; Pineapple Cherry-licious Explosion, **174**

Pineapple Cherry-licious Explosion, **174**

pizza: Almond Butter and Jelly Breakfast Pizza, **154**; Little Lunch Box Mini Pizzas, **210**

Poached Eggs with Honey Mustard Spinach, **152**

Polenta, Grilled Chicken and Shiitake Mushrooms with, **192**

Polish study, 120–121

polypeptides, 45

popcorn, 87, 137

Portobello Steaks, **225**

positive lifestyle changes, *x*, 28–29

Positive Options for Living with Your Ostomy (White), 17

potassium, 104

Potato, Bacon, and Arugula Hash, **162**

potatoes, 89, 102; Nourishing Potato Soup, **185**; Oven-Roasted Chicken and Potatoes, **200**; Pepper and Potato Hash, **158**; Potato, Bacon, and Arugula Hash, **162**; Sweet Potato Muffins, **182**; Sweet Potato Pancakes, **147**; Sweet Potato Strudel, **150**

poultry, 145, 191; Apple Rosemary Cornish Game Hens, **194–195**. *See also* chicken; turkey

Primary Health Puzzle Pieces (PHPPs), 17–19, 50

probiotics, 11; antibiotics *vs.*, 119–120; bacteria and, 37, 82, 119–120; benefits of, 120–121; how to take, 121; purchasing, 121

processed foods, overconsumption of, *ix*, 14

proctocolectomy, 16

prostacyclin, 128

protease, 46, 123

proteins: daily requirements, 109–110; food intolerances and, 4, 45, 46–47; signs of inadequate, 110; in vegetarian and vegan diet, 109–111

pudding: Brown Rice Pudding, **245**; Mock Cook 'n' Serve Vanilla Pudding, **246**

Pumped-Up Piña Colada Smoothie, **167**

pumpkin: Pumpkin Pie Healthy Egg Cream, **172**; Pumpkin Quinoa Cookies, **234–235**

Pumpkin Pie Healthy Egg Cream, **172**

Pumpkin Quinoa Cookies, **234–235**

Q

quinoa, 107, 110; Lemon and Basil Quinoa, **212**; Pumpkin Quinoa Cookies, **234–235**

R

Rasio, Debora, 25

reintroduction diet, 65–68; guidelines for, 66–67; physical and emotional balance and, 67; physical and emotional symptoms and, 67–68; results of, 68; sample reintroduction chart, 68

rice: Dairy-Free Whipped Rice Cream, **243**; Grilled Asparagus, Rice, and Peas, **220**; Very Vanilla Rice Milk, **170**. *See also* brown rice

Rice Noodles in Basil Butter Sauce, **215**

Roasted Carrots with Molasses and Dill, **222**

Roasted Cauliflower and White Wine Pasta, **214**

Roasted Garlic Hummus, **189**

Roasted Lemon Broccoli, **217**

rotation diet, 49, 59, 69–71; example of, 70–71; rules, 69–70
Round-Up Ready (RUR), 87–88
Rubin, Jordan, 3, 4, 36
RUR. *See* Round-Up Ready

S

salads: Carrot and Raisin Salad, **227**; Cheerfully Cherry Pecan Salad, **229**; Far-Out Fruit Salad, **228**; Kiwi Avocado Salad, **231**; Mango-Strawberry Salad, **232**; Tangy Tuna Salad, **230**; Tomato and Pasta Salad, **208**
salmon: Grilled Salmon with Honey Ginger Sauce, **204**; Our Favorite Salmon, **206**
salt, 144
saturated fats, 123
sauces. *See* dressings, sauces, and dips
sauerkraut, 105
Screw its, 141
seafood. *See* fish and seafood
serotonin, 21, 55
Sesame Glazed Ginger Tuna Steaks with Brown Rice, **207**
shellfish, 46
Shrimp, Baked Coconut, **205**
Sicko (documentary), 21
Side Effects Bible (Vagnini), 27
Simple Grilled Chicken, **191**
Simple Roasted Swiss Chard, **218**
Simple Watermelon Chiller, **171**
Simply Classic Lemon Pepper Rosemary Chicken, **202**
Simply Simple Avocado Dip, **251**
Slow Cook Beef Tender, **201**
Smith, Dorothy, 25
smoking, 14
smoothies, 104, 105, 163–164, 166–167, 169
snacks and desserts, 233–247
soups, 183–186
soy: substitutes and avoiding, 79–80; as top allergen, 46
Spaghetti Squash, Summery, **221**
Specific Carbohydrate Diet (Gottschall), 36
Spinach, Poached Eggs with Honey Mustard, **152**
Stephanie's story, 8–11, 34–35

steroids, 3; long-term use of, 26
Steve's story, 81–83
stevia, 93
strawberries: Cranberry Strawberry Breakfast Bars, **157**; Mango-Strawberry Salad, **232**; Strawberry Cranberry Smoothie, **164**
Strawberry Cranberry Smoothie, **164**
stress: in case study, 52–53, 55–56; impacts of, 10, 18, 34, 45, 96; oxidative stress, 117–118; ruling out, 2; stress hormones, 45, 97; treatment for, 11, 17
sucrose, 90
sugar, 90–97; alternative names for, 91, 93; amount consumed per year, 90; beating addiction to, 91–93, 100–101; quiz, 93–97. *See also* natural sweeteners
Summery Spaghetti Squash, **221**
Sun-Dried Tomato Grilled Eggplant, **224**
Super Baby Foods (Yaron), 105
supplements, 115–128; benefits of, 117–118; negative interactions from, 118; recommended, 5, 26, 50, 108, 119–128; survey, 119; types commonly used, 119. *See also* vitamins; *specific supplements*
surgery, 12, 16–17
Swedish study, 91
Sweet Collard Green Stuffing, **219**
sweeteners, natural, 92–93, 233
sweet potatoes: Oven-Roasted Chicken and Potatoes, **200**; Sweet Potato Muffins, **182**; Sweet Potato Pancakes, **147**; Sweet Potato Strudel, **150**
Sweet Potato Muffins, **182**
Sweet Potato Pancakes, **147**
Sweet Potato Strudel, **150**
Swiss Chard, Simple Roasted, **218**
sympathetic nervous system (fight-or-flight system), 44

T

Tangy Tuna Salad, **230**
tea, 99
Teeccino, 99
tests: blood testing, 49, 58–63, 83; for Crohn's disease, 1, 4; for food

intolerances, 10, 32, 37, 47–50, 52–56; urine test, 116
Tiffany's story, 129–130
Tofu Sour Cream, Totally, 248
Tomato and Pasta Salad, 208
tomatoes, 102; Falafel Nuggets with Tomato Sauce, 176–177; Sun-Dried Tomato Grilled Eggplant, 224; Tomato and Pasta Salad, 208; Tomato Simmered String Beans, 226; 20-Minute Tomato Soup, 183
Tomato Simmered String Beans, 226
Totally Tofu Sour Cream, 248
Transformation Enzyme Products, 265
Triad Profile, 49, 263
trisaccharides, 187
Tudor-Locke, Catrine, 19
tuna: Sesame Glazed Ginger Tuna Steaks with Brown Rice, 207; Tangy Tuna Salad, 230
turkey: Curry Turkey Tenders, 197; Orange Marmalade Turkey Burgers, 196
turmeric, 127
20-Minute Tomato Soup, 183

U
Un-French Onion Soup, 186
urine test, 116
USDA food pyramid, 85–86
USDA MyPlate, 83–86

V
Vagnini, Frederick, 27
vanilla: Homemade Vanilla Almond Milk, 168; Mock Cook 'n' Serve Vanilla Pudding, 246; Very Vanilla Rice Milk, 170
vegetables, 102–106, 216–226; Chicken and Veggie Tacos, 193; eating more, 91–92; for flare-ups, 103–106; leafy, green, 103–104, 145, 216; Mexican Fiesta Rice 'n' Beans with Veggies, 190; Nana's Vegetable Dip, 249; puréed, 104–105, 233. See also specific vegetables
vegetarian and vegan diet, 108–111
Very Vanilla Rice Milk, 170
villi, 13, 47

Virgin Piña Colada Smoothie Pops, 236
vitamins, 116–117; B vitamins, 108–109, 124–125; deficiencies, 108, 118; eating more, 89; multivitamin, 126; in vegetarian and vegan diet, 108–109; vitamin C, 118, 126, 144

W
Waffles, Wonderful Blueberry Walnut, 156
Wareham, Ellsworth, 24
water: drinking, 91, 95, 163; protecting supply of, 88–89
Watermelon Chiller, Simple, 171
websites: eatwellguide.org, 145; Environmental Working Group, 144–145; Healthnotes, 118; Metametrix Clinical Laboratory, 49, 263; for nutritional data, 143; Teeccino, 99
Weil, Andrew, 101
Western medicine common treatment methods, 15–17
What Are Your Top Three Health Goals?, 18, 33–34
wheat: substitutes and avoiding, 77–78; as top allergen, 46
Wheel of Digestive Health, 18, 29, 35, 50
White, Craig A., 17
white foods, 86, 92
WHO. See World Health Organization
Winfrey, Oprah, 29
Wonder Laboratories, 266
Wonderful Blueberry Walnut Waffles, 156
words of wisdom, 140–141
World Health Organization (WHO), 22
World Journal of Gastroenterology, 12
Wrap, Blissful Breakfast, 160

Y
Yaron, Ruth, 105
yogurt: Granola and Yogurt Parfait, 153; substitutions for, 74
you are what you eat, ix, 19
Yummy, Healthy Onion Rings, 237

Z
Zesty Zucchini or Eggplant Sticks, 238–239